CORE EXERCISES FOR SENIORS

Daily Activities to Build Balance, Strength, and Confidence

Stanford Dyson

CONTENTS

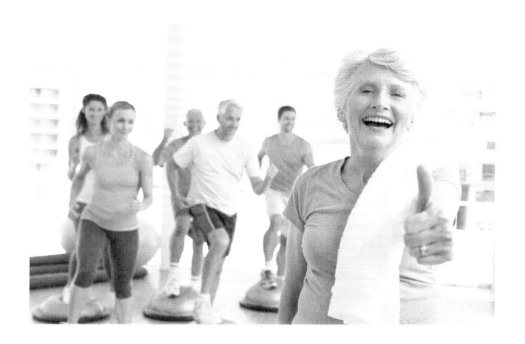

INTRODUCTION

Congratulations on purchasing *Core exercises for seniors,* and thank you for doing so.

The following chapters will discuss the different means of strengthening your core muscles in detail. The first and foremost step to staying young even after growing old is practicing self-love and self-care. You and your strength or capability to do every single task on your own matter the most. It's always lovely to stay independent. Are you looking for ways of becoming older with grace and vitality? Chances are there that you might not be sure about the correct ways of achieving that. You need not worry as you are in the right place, which means you have the hunger for attaining information and also the willingness to learn more for a better senior life. In this practical and instructional guide, learning about the most effective pillar of lively and enthusiastic aging, i.e., a toned and strong core, will help you greatly.

This book will assist seniors in realizing that core exercises and fitness are one of the most effective transformative tools to heal their body, mind, and spirit. Besides healing, such a fitness tool also plays a preventive role so that your body does not face further decline. In this book, we will discuss in detail about advantages of strengthening your core, signs of identifying that your core is weak, myths of exercises that seniors must avoid, standing and seating core exercises, benefits of choosing an exercise partner, ways of getting relief from pains and aches, foods for a stronger core, etc. Once you reach the last part of this book on core exercises for senior citizens, you will definitely get the necessary tools for moving confidently with a firm and powerful core.

There are plenty of books on this subject on the market, thanks again for choosing this one! Every effort was made to ensure it is full of as much useful information as possible. *Please enjoy!*

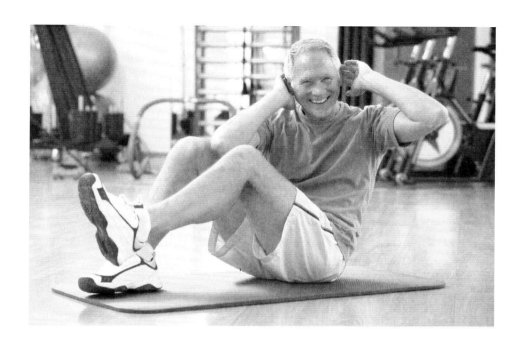

CHAPTER 1: YOUR BODY, AGING, AND CORE

Age – Well, it is nothing other than just a number! How many of you think in this manner? It is true to some extent as it is always better to stay and feel young from both mind and heart. But, you cannot ignore the fact of aging altogether, especially when the matter is about the various changes that occur in your body because of increased age. You cannot avoid age, whereas it is possible to avoid aging. Growing old is one of the basic elements of life. Usually, a person is labeled as old when they hit the age bar of 60. This thought was true in the past times as life span was shorter, and surviving even after 60 years was unusual then. But at present, older individuals tend to live their lives actively even after stepping into the seventh and eighth decades of their life.

The strength and physical abilities of a 65-year-old person may vary a lot from another whose age is nearly 80 years. Such variation depends on their fitness level, overall health, and mental awareness. Other than the age factor, various other aspects also lead to such differences, including regular exercise, food habits, lifestyle, adequate sleep, body weight, and enriching activities. It is impossible to control your chronological age, but controlling your biological age is possible by the options you choose. To comprehend this matter in a better manner, here is a simple example for you. Think of a man whose age is nearly 70 years and who suffered breast cancer. After completing his struggle, he chooses a diet containing fresh fruits, lean proteins, fresh vegetables, etc. Besides this, he even practices regular stretching exercises to strengthen his muscles and stay fit and flexible, solves jigsaw puzzles daily, and also plays golf thrice a week. Now, think of another man of the same age who does not suffer from any major health issues except very minute arthritis in his hands. He opts for processed foods rich in sugar and salt. Not only does he consume an unhealthy diet, but he also avoids regular core exercise and spends most of the time sitting idle or watching television. If you look from the chronological point of view, both of them belong to the same age. But the rate of their biological aging is different.

When a person's age increases by numbers, they get the blessings of immense wisdom, an ample amount of family time, opportunities to travel more frequently, etc. Is there anyone who is not fond of senior discounts? Besides all such benefits, senior individuals do face certain physical challenges. As your age elevates, your body starts declining gradually. Your memory starts to weaken, and you force your mind a lot to recall thoughts or memories that you once found easier to remember. Your overall metabolism begins to diminish as well as your body balance falters. The bones start shrinking, and thus the risk of fractures increases a lot.

The various symptoms related to aging might be quite frustrating, but there is always a way out. Fighting Osteoporosis and preventing bones from breaking will become easier by following a daily exercise routine. It is necessary to prepare yourself for dealing with the difficulties of old age as it will assist you in staying mentally and physically strong. Senior individuals will be able to stay steady on their feet as well as heal from falls quickly if they practice stability and balance moves. Other than recovering more rapidly, moving the body is also helpful in releasing physical and mental stress and keeping the brain sharp even in old age. Regular exercises are also beneficial in letting your metabolism function more efficiently. You will find it exciting when you are able to button your favorite trousers a bit easier.

By going through this chapter, you will get a brief knowledge about the changes that happen in your body as you grow by numbers. Other than that, you will also get information about your core muscles.

First of all, you need to realize that your body does not renew in the same manner as it did when you were younger. The cellular turnover starts declining with age; in other words, a person starts losing both bone density and muscle mass. Usually, cells undergo remodeling, and muscles and bones regenerate more when broken down at young age. But the number of regeneration decreases as an individual ages. Usually, muscle cells possess self-renewal capacity. With increased age, a person's body does not build as much muscle and bone. The sad part is that you won't get back cent percent of what you have lost from your body unless you train it accordingly. Losing bone density and balance is a dangerous combination; thus, falling down is one of the major risk factors as you age. Feeling worried about how you will deal with the changes you will face due to aging? Here is some good news for you. You will be able to safeguard your body balance and keep your muscles strong by building a strong core. It is impossible to possess a smooth balance without a stable core. It's just that simple!

Can you swing your gold club swiftly, or cut the hedge of your lawn shorter, or enjoy kayaking? If you can do such activities requiring sufficient movement, then you must be grateful and thank your core. Having healthy and active core muscles is an essential part of your health and overall well-being. Besides this, core muscles also play a vital role in keeping a person stable and mobile. Your stability will ensure that you get to do your tasks without other people's assistance as you grow older. This, in turn, is helpful in keeping a person self-dependent for a longer time span. Core muscles are also helpful in regulating your bladder and breathing function.

Do you remember the last time when you felt excited about exercising for your midsection? Getting a negative response regarding this matter will not at all be surprising. On the other hand, if you switch your thoughts from a workout to its effects, you will realize that getting delighted about core fitness is worth it. Various reliable surveys, including seniors, state that one of the leading concerns related to aging is giving importance to physical fitness. The secret to attaining physical freedom is by maintaining core strength. You will start enjoying the effects only after you include core exercises in your regular schedule. The first response that you will feel is better control of your balance and a greater extent of motion. Gradually, you will start feeling comfortable and confident in whatever attire you put on.

Now, let's look to get an in-depth idea of what core is. A maximum number of individuals hold a belief that the core only involves the abdominal muscles. Whereas it is something more than that. Your abdominal muscles are indeed an integral part of your core. But the torso girdle is made up of almost 35 muscles that support your body. Truly speaking, your core is a complex network of nerves, bones, tendons, ligaments, and every single muscle that is connected to the spine. All these elements wrap the entire body as well as extend downwards beneath the hips. Core muscles are highly essential for maintaining a proper balance within your pelvis, kinetic chain, and spine. Strong core muscles are helpful in protecting your spine from the enormous load and transferring excessive load between your lower and upper body. Here is a list of the major core muscles:

Obliques stretch diagonally, starting from the ribs to the pelvis, and this particular core muscle contains two sets, namely, internal oblique muscles and external oblique muscles. The external set is located just over the internal oblique muscles. The muscle fiber in every single group runs perpendicular to each other. Both the set of muscles work as a single unit and help rotate your torso, bend your torso side by side, and round your spine. Twisting and turning your body is the main function of obliques. These muscles also enable in supporting your spine whenever you lift any heavy object.

The Rectus abdominis is one of the vital core muscles, which is thought of as 'six-pack muscles' by a huge number of people. These muscles are present vertically along both sides of the abdomen, starting from your sternum towards the pubic bone. The Rectus abdominis plays a great role in tilting your pelvis and also in letting people bend their torso in the forward direction.

The transverse abdominis is another major core muscle located just in the front part of a person's body, on both sides of the navel. These muscles are stratified just beneath the oblique muscles. The transverse abdominis is known to be the innermost abdominal muscle. These core muscles enable an individual to breathe and play a vital role in stabilizing your pelvis and lower spine while you move.

The Gluteus maximus is the next core muscle that is located inside your buttocks. By its location, it is easy to understand that these core muscles help an individual to walk and climb stairs. Gluteus maximus turns out to be helpful when a person tries to lift his/her legs.

Erector spinae core muscles are present on both sides of the vertebral column. These muscles are known to extend by the side of your spine's thoracic, cervical, and lumbar sections. The function of erector spinae muscles is to straighten your back and let you stand upright. You can rotate your body from one side to the other because of these core muscles. Usually, a person suffers from back pain and spasms if a strain or injury affects these muscles.

Transversospinalis is a group of core muscles that run along your spine, from your head to your pelvis. This muscle group plays the role of stabilizing your vertebral column as well as enabling spinal movement. The core muscles along your spine help maintain your balance even at those times when you are not consciously thinking about your balance. Thus, transversospinalis lets you remain aware of your body's position.

Latissimus dorsi often termed 'lats,' are the largest muscles in the upper portion of your body. This group of muscles runs all across the back side of your body, starting from beneath the shoulder blades straight down to the pelvis. This core muscle helps in moving your shoulders and also in stabilizing your spine.

The above-mentioned brief overview will help you in getting an idea about the functions of the vital core muscles. Apart from these muscles, various other core muscles are also present inside your body that are also helpful in supporting your body in some way or the other. By now, you might have understood that core strength is more than gaining the capability to do a hundred sit-ups. It is a systematic phenomenon for preventing injuries and also for relieving pain. Your core muscles support your spine, and if the supporting muscles are weak, the other essential groups of muscles need to compensate. If such a situation arises, your entire body's alignment will get disturbed, along with increased pain in your hips, knees, and backside. In such circumstances, the tendency to lose body balance also gets elevated.

The strength of your core muscles, especially in the abdominal region, is necessary for bringing yourself up from a seated position to a standing one. If you find out that you have to rely on your arms and hands to push yourself up, it is simply because your core is not strong enough to pull yourself up. A lot of factors may lead to balance issues. But in most cases, it is because of the deficiency of stability in core muscles. Core muscles are helpful in stabilizing a person when they turn, twist, walk, or go through any sort of movement. No matter which core exercises you practice, be it modified plank or straight arm, it is the responsibility of your core to keep your backside straight during exercises. If you notice that any part of your lower body is sagging, then you need to identify that sign as a failure of your core to perform its duties.

Now, it's time to move to the next chapter, where we will get to know certain information about a weak core.

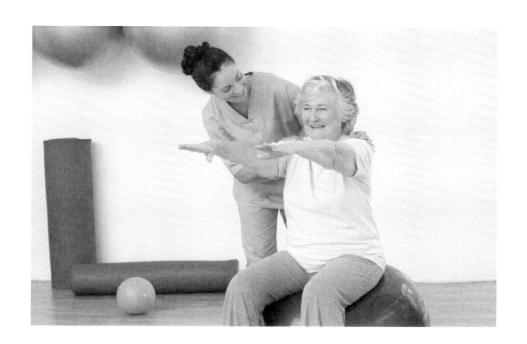

CHAPTER 2: SIGNS TO IDENTIFY THAT YOU HAVE A WEAK CORE

The core is something that helps a person stay upright as well as lets them stay strong in their daily posture. If your core is working properly and strong, you will definitely have better posture, lesser back pain, and enjoy the movement of the various body parts with more endurance and ease. Can you imagine the huge amount of problems that you will face if your core muscles fall weak? Of course, you can. Now the question that might arise in your mind is how will you know whether your core is strong or weak? Many individuals think that a thin waist, chiseled abs, or ability to do uncountable sit-ups at a time are signs of possessing a healthy and strong core. Whereas the truth is something different. All these signs are not reliable to let you understand the actual strength of your core. Here in this chapter, we will talk about the various signs to identify that you have a weak core.

But before that, let's go through a few questions which might enable you to test the strength of your core. While going through the questions, you need to be honest with your answers. You need not worry as nobody is going to judge your abilities. Have a look at the questions:

Do you frequently feel that your lower back is hurting or becoming stiff, notably after exercise? (Yes/No)
Do you hold your breath unintentionally during exercise? (Yes/No)
Can you lift up a foot from the floor by keeping your eyes closed and maintaining your body balance? (Yes/No)
Suppose you are sitting on a chair or on the floor. Can you stand erect without using your arms or hands? (Yes/No)
Does your lower back or midsection drop down while you hold the plank position? (Yes/No)

If you replied affirmatively to a minimum number of two questions, then for sure, it is time to strengthen your core.

To check your core's strength, you may also perform a few easy tests, for example, the hollowing test or the plank test. While performing the hollowing test, you first need to sit down comfortably. Once you are comfortable in your position, start inhaling and exhaling. While breathing out, you must try pulling your stomach towards your spine for somewhat ten seconds. If you are unable to stay in this position for the mentioned time, that will serve as an indication that your core muscles are weak. You may also go for the plank test. For this, you need to stay in the position of doing pushups. Your entire body weight must remain rested on your arms, toes, and elbows. Pay attention to your hip, as it must be steady and level. If you fail to remain in such a position for at least forty to fifty seconds, it will give you the indication that your core is weak.

Now, let's move to the following part, where you will get information about a few common signs that will let you know that your core strength is insufficient.

Having Poor Balance

Whether you believe it or not, your ankles and feet are not the only body parts that assist you in balancing. The strength of your core muscles plays a great role here. Though there are various reasons behind suffering from a poor balance, the weak core is one of the major culprits. The core muscles are helpful in stabilizing the pelvis. You will enjoy good body balance only if your pelvis is stable. Your balance will be affected if your glutes and hip muscles surrounding your pelvis are weak. The bad balance will not protect you from falls. The stability provided by core muscles lets a person move in all possible directions, most importantly on irregular terrains. Core muscles also keep on working even when you are standing in a spot and thus prevent you from collapsing. It is not always possible to notice this problem of poor balance from the very beginning. To realize whether your ability to maintain body balance is suffering or not, all you need to do is perform one or more tests. For checking your balance, stand erect by keeping one foot on the floor and the other off the floor. You need to close your eyes during this balance-checking test. Once you are done with one foot, repeat the same with the other one. If you are able to stay in this position for a minimum time of ten seconds, then your core strength is somewhat okay. But if you cannot do so, you will get to understand that your balance is suffering, and probabilities are there that it is because of your underdeveloped or weak core.

Having Lower Back Pain

Have you ever felt a pinch, twinge, or tweak while performing your regular movements, such as taking out a bowl from the oven, tossing a toy to your pet dog, or handling your laundry? If yes, it's time for you to blame the strength of your core muscles. If your core is not strong enough as it must be, the lumbar spine may become shaky. This, in turn, puts unnecessary pressure on your discs, vertebrae, and other muscles which enclose the spine. One of the most common signs of possessing reduced core stability is struggling with lower back pain. Core muscles work together to stabilize your trunk and your spine. Thus, your must not neglect your lower back pain at all. It might be a severe indication of weak core muscles.

The pain can be mild as well as acute, and it all depends on how severe your condition is. Weaker muscle strength fails to give you the required support to your vertebrae and discs, giving rise to pain and discomfort. Usually, the lower back possesses a forward curve. But achieving this curved position will be impossible if the core muscles are not strong enough. It leads to pain in the tendons and surrounding muscles. If the core muscles are not conditioned properly, your spine will face the risk of being overworked, and you will not be able to avoid tension and muscular strain. Consequently, you will start feeling the side effects of excessive stress on the lower back portion of your body. Other than that, you may also feel such pain in the neck region. You will find simple activities such as lifting something, walking, and bending totally miserable.

Having Poor Posture

Healthy posture is essential for the overall well-being of your bladder, bowler, and spine. Besides this, it is also necessary for proper breathing. Whether you will have a good or poor posture depends entirely on the strength of your core. If you possess a weak core, you will start to slump or slouch more. To check your posture, you must simply stand straight in front of a mirror and start checking your profile. It will assist you in observing the way you stand. You may also go for another option. Ask any close friend of yours or your family member to click your picture in the standing position both from the side and front. Observe your pictures carefully. If you notice that the position of your head is just above the shoulders and the upper portion of your shoulders over your hips, then you have a good posture. Your tissues will feel less stressed, and the chances of you suffering from pain will be less if all your body parts are in alignment.

But if you do not notice the required alignment, then sorry to state that your posture is poor, and you need to work on your core stability. Weak core muscles fail to provide sufficient stability to the pelvis and the spine, which results in a bad posture. An increased level of discomfort and a lot of complications may arise if you do not pay attention to your posture and leave it unattended.

Your Wrists and Feet Hurt

Nowadays, a large number of people complain about wrist pain or foot pain. Such pain keeps returning even after undergoing physical therapy or any other effective treatment. When your core strength is weak and there is a lack of stability and adequate central support, your joints and outer muscles will ultimately suffer. You have already learned about the necessity of proper balance, especially when a person starts growing older. When your core fails to work properly and thus does not assist you in staying more stable, all the pressure will fall on your feet. In such situations, your feet will have to take up the responsibility of working harder. It will result in giving trouble to the tissues present on your foot's bottom side. On the other hand, if you do not receive sufficient support from the middle back portion while pulling or pushing something, your elbows and wrists will take the burden. This may give rise to pain or stiffness of your wrist over time. Getting hurt on your wrists and feet may be one common indication of having a weak core.

Struggle Getting Up or Down

Pay close attention to your body movements when you try standing up from a chair or bed. Did you find it difficult to stand up? Did you take the help of your hands or arms while getting up? If you observe that you need to hold the handles of your chair to push yourself down from a standing position or while trying to sit, your legs and core may require strengthening. While standing erect from a lying or sitting position, an unreliable amount of core strength is necessary. Besides depending on core muscles, you also need to depend on your glutes and abs to support your body. If your core muscles possess poor strength in those particular areas, your body will try to take the support from elsewhere, like your arms, to receive that power. Whereas, if you notice that getting up from the chair or sitting down can be done with ease without utilizing your arms, then your core muscles are strong and fit.

Always Holding Breath

Do you always need someone to remind you to breathe while doing exercise or moving? If yes, that indicates that you possess a weak core that is not working appropriately. The diaphragm is the major breathing muscle. If there is a lack of stability in your core, the main breathing muscle will start contracting in order to compensate. One of the most common signs to understand that your diaphragm is trying to make up for the instability of core muscles is holding your breath always during exercise. Though it is one of the common tell-tale signs, it is also one of the most unnoticed signs of a weak core. Correcting this particular problem is actually a bit difficult. For this, you need to start breathing every single moment, as it will prevent your diaphragm from staying contracted.

Difficulty to Stand for a Long Period

Is there anybody who loves to stand in long queues? Most probably, every single individual hates to do so. But suppose you prefer avoiding long lines as it is seriously intolerable for you to keep standing for a lengthy period. In that case, you might need to practice some endurance or strength exercises. Some people think that their muscles work only when they remain active. But the truth is something different. Core muscles do not stop working under any condition throughout your entire life. These muscles are critical when your body is in an erect position. Thus, if you notice that you are finding it difficult to keep yourself in an upright position for an extended period, take it as an indication of weak core muscles.

Feeling Weak While Jumping or Throwing

Did you ever feel weak while performing certain exercises, such as tossing a heavy ball, jumping continuously, hitting a punch, or doing a bicep curl? Some of you might not face any difficulty while doing such activities. Whereas many are there who will find it tough to do the above-mentioned activities. If you fall in the second category, it means that your core muscles are not properly trained. Core muscles have the responsibility of stabilizing and sending power and giving strength to various other muscles. If you do not possess the required strength in your midline, your distal parts, including your legs, arms, ankles, or shoulders, will not be strong enough.

Thus, maintaining a fit and healthy body is possible if your core strength is sufficient. Your whole body is affected whenever your muscles begin losing the required strength. If your core is weak, lifting up things of minimal weight will become difficult for you. Weak core muscles make a person feel tired and weak even after doing regular and small work. Such difficulties will increase with age. By now, you might have become aware of your core strength. It's time to learn about the benefits of strengthening your core muscles. You will gain the motivation to give importance to your core muscles after knowing those advantages. *Please, turn the page!*

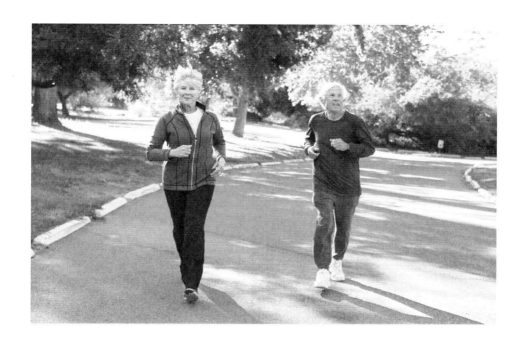

CHAPTER 3: ADVANTAGES OF STRENGTHENING YOUR CORE MUSCLES

Everything we do in our daily life, from standing upright to walking confidently, sitting down to reaching, we always depend on our muscles to keep us steady or moving boldly. A lot of individuals do not give a second thought to those essential muscles. When the matter is about your core muscles, you must keep them flexible and fit as it will enable you to upgrade your healthy life. While bending down to tie up your shoelace, stretching your arms to reach out to a glass kept on the shelf, or cleaning the floor, in all such cases, you are actually utilizing your core muscles—almost all sorts of movements that you do regularly require core stability. No matter which part of your body starts moving, it ripples downward and upward to the adjacent core muscles. Thus, an inflexible or weak core may impair the functioning power of your legs and arms.

Not only is strengthening your core muscles advantageous for your physical appearance, but it also serves as a major factor for your overall body balance, health, and performance during exercises. Being an essential link between your lower and upper body, your core plays the role of a dictator for dictating various ways of doing your daily activities. A strong and stable core is necessary for effective movement. Many individuals hold a confusion regarding what core is, and so they think that working on your core muscles is simply performing ab workouts. It is actually something more than that. Making your core strong means training your back and hips, along with learning different ways of stabilizing the muscles.

By strengthening your core muscles, you will be able to do your daily tasks more quickly and enhance your overall well-being. This chapter will teach you about certain benefits of strengthening your core muscles.

Improves Posture

Do you know that your spine undergoes wear and tear on a regular basis? You will be able to decrease the impact of such wear and tear by possessing a good posture. How is it possible to attain a good posture? Well, the answer is you will be able to improve your posture by strengthening your core muscles. A well-defined posture is also helpful in letting you breathe better than ever before by making sure that the life-saving gas is reaching your muscles adequately. Your core wraps the entire torso region, which includes all the muscles present in your back and sides. So, when the core is healthier, especially the inner muscles, it assists in attaining an improved posture.

By making your core strong, your spine's position will become straightened. It will also assist in stretching the back portion of your body so that you can align the posture appropriately. Besides this, a stronger core and good posture help in preventing a few irritating back and neck pain that arises because of bending over the computer or laptop regularly. In today's hectic life, almost every individual spends a maximum part of the day doing desk work. Sitting in this manner for a long time and that too regularly negatively impacts the strength of your core muscles. If you follow a similar work situation, you must take short breaks between the long sit and work periods and utilize the breaks by stretching or walking casually.

Enhances Stability

Many experts state that possessing a stout and powerful torso enables a person to stay steady irrespective of the activity they do. Stronger core muscles engage the hips, pelvis, and lower back for better collaboration and provide both stability and balance to the entire body. Being stable does not mean staying on your feet and preventing falls. It is necessary to strengthen your core muscles as you will find it easier to stand straighter. It will also help you stabilize your trunk during daily activities and even workouts. The chances of suffering from lower back pain, poor posture, and muscle injuries will heighten if you have weaker core muscles. Regular activities like running, sitting, and walking can be performed more efficiently by strengthening your core and enhancing stability. It is because the alignment of your body will improve with the increased strength of your core. Moreover, the strain you could feel on your joints and muscles also starts reducing.

Makes Daily Life Easier

The foundation of all the movements of your daily life is your core. It is necessary to strengthen your core to execute your regular movements, such as bending to pick up something from the ground, performing various household chores, or standing for a long time in a better and easier manner. The stronger your core is, the more convenient it will be for you to lead your daily life. Thus, various core exercises that are meant for seniors are under the category of functional fitness. Such workouts enable aged people to lead their day more functionally and with more ease. So start strengthening your core muscles to enjoy the benefit of an easier and smoother daily life.

Prevents or Reduces Pain

Are you willing to know one more vital perk of having a healthy core? A strong core will assist you in feeling better overall. One of the best benefits of strengthening your core muscles is that it will enhance the quality of your life. Most importantly, it will decrease as well as prevent any sort of pain that you might be suffering from. Besides this, a well-developed core also helps strengthen the spine, supports the lower back, and much more. It is true that exercise comes last on the list when you suffer from chronic pain. Whereas many reliable studies praise the advantages of core strength workouts for reducing hip and back pain. Although the causes of chronic back pain are numerous, experienced researchers are aware of the fact that there exists a relation between weak core muscles, issues related to mobility, and the intensity of back pain.

Better posture and balance, moving around easily, etc., are those benefits of a strong core that enable you to avoid irritation and diminish the discomfort that you face due to habits like sitting in front of computers the entire day. A strong core will decrease your body pain and discomfort and let you feel your best. If you possess an upright and aligned body, the pain and back injuries will gradually decrease. By now, you are already aware that the core supports your back, neck, spine, and muscles. If you follow core exercises to strengthen your core muscles, the pressure on your back muscles will reduce. Besides this, you will also be able to work harder to decrease muscle strains, support your body, and decrease the chances of back pain and injury.

Protects Some of Your Organs

Being a living organism, you are very well aware of the fact that organs play a major role in the proper functioning of your body. Strong core muscles may assist you by keeping a few of your vital organs safe. Various organs, such as your spleen, liver, kidneys, etc., are located just below your abdominal wall; this, in turn, acts as a protector against the outer world. Thus, the stronger core you have, the better it will protect your tissues from external damage or force of any type. Isn't this benefit of strengthening your core muscles quite interesting? *So, start working on it!*

Improves Body Balance

The next advantage of well-maintained core strength along with enhanced posture is enjoying a gradual improvement in your body balance. A lot of people complain of an occasional trip or stumble in their regular life. But you must not be surprised about it as such a stumble does not cause any danger to your regular life. Whereas some individuals are there who consume specific medications or try to manage health conditions like arthritis. Usually, such people tend to suffer from balance and coordination problems regularly. One more factor for having poor balance is nothing other than aging. Numerous reliable studies state that seniors who follow regular core strength-enhancing exercises report enjoying improved independence, balance, and quality of their lives.

Stronger core muscles will lead to better body balance, consisting of muscles that tend to work together to support your body. Not only will you find it beneficial in improving the balance of your body parts, but it will also reduce the strain present in your joints and muscles. The risk of getting injured will also get minimized. A strong core has the ability to create equilibrium inside your body. It will even enable you to stand for a longer time than ever before and also develop a balance all through your physical being.

Enhances Flexibility

To understand this particular benefit of strengthening your core muscles, here is a brief description of a reliable study examining the outcome or impact of one month's core strength training program. In this study, the participants were active students who were divided into two control and training groups. Students who were the training group members performed several exercises for about half an hour each day at a stretch of five days every week. They performed those exercises which involved movements targeting the multifidus, transverse abdominis, muscles of the pelvic floor, and diaphragm to escalate their spine's stability. After following the same routine for four weeks, the researchers analyzed that the core stability of the training group exhibited desirable effects.

From the findings of such trustworthy studies, various experts suggest that other than young people, even older adults may receive benefits by performing targeted core workouts. Such exercises help in improving movement control as well as posture reaction. Once you learn ways of engaging your core, it will assist you in staying upright before any fall or injury. Flexibility is all that matters for the proper movement of your body parts.

Improves Performance

The next advantage of making your core strong is enhancing your performance, be it related to sports or regular workouts. By now, almost all of you know that a toned and healthy core improves stability, and stability is highly essential during workouts. Having a strong core is also helpful in better synchronization of your upper body and legs while you play sports or perform exercises. You will also find it easier to perform heavy movements resulting in less stress on your muscles. Several studies have been done in the past years related to core training for athletes, especially runners. In one such reliable study, male athletes from college underwent a core training program for almost eight weeks. The participants revealed the benefits that because of strengthening their core muscles, they enjoyed an improvement in endurance, energy level while running, and static balance.

While running, core muscles present in the glutes, back, hips, and spine are engaged. Thus, possibilities are there that following certain core exercises meant for various target muscles may benefit older adults in improving their running or jogging speed, form, and, most importantly, their respiration. Having a strong core is helpful in sustaining solid form while you run. Strengthening your core muscles will not let you spend excess energy as the muscles of your pelvic, hips, etc., will start working more smoothly. If you practice core exercises regularly, you will get an opportunity to avoid injury or strain while jogging or running for miles.

Burns Fat

Did you just smile out of excitement after going through this particular advantage of strengthening your core? Quite obviously, many individuals will feel the urge to strengthen their core muscles after knowing that it helps burn excessive fat. Toning and core strengthening exercises are an outstanding way of quickly burning your abdominal, leg, and side fat. To make your core strong, you need to follow core exercises on a regular basis. Core exercises involve practicing ballistic movements, which combine flexibility, cardio, and strength training. This, in turn, helps build strength and become lean by burning fat.

If you increase your core strength, you will get a lot better support to try out various forms of workouts. By prioritizing the strength of your core, you will provide your body with a firm foundation for the remaining parts of your body. It even includes an enhanced ability to perform weight-bearing workouts correctly. An active and healthy lifestyle is an essential element of growing older, and such a lifestyle can be well-maintained by strengthening your core. Every single individual wishes to survive independently without anybody's assistance. Core strength enables an individual to keep themselves mobile as they age, so increasing their strength will let them age well.

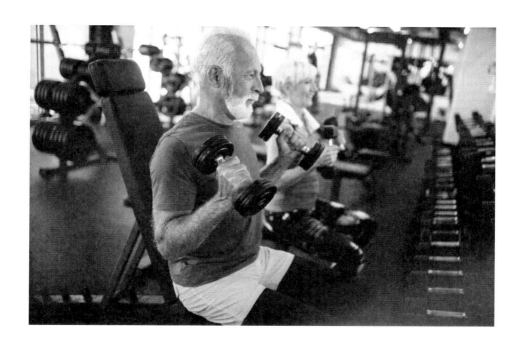

CHAPTER 4: WHEN AND WHERE TO EXERCISE YOUR CORE?

Remaining stable and strong is an integral factor of aging properly. Suppose you wish to dwell a fulfilling, interesting, and active life even after entering your sixties, eighties, and ahead. In that case, it is necessary to retain your abilities to perform regular tasks. Maintaining your core strength and remaining physically active are vital for all the activities you enjoy even after you grow older. You need to perform regular core exercises to enjoy your senior citizenship days. When the matter is about doing workouts, many people have a lot of questions to ask as well, as a huge number of confusions revolve around their minds. One of the most common dilemmas that almost every individual comes across is when is the best or perfect time to exercise the core. Is your name also on this list of people who face such confusion? If yes, then you are certainly in the right place at this moment.

To know when and where to exercise your core, all you need to do is just keep reading ahead. Hopefully, you will get all the necessary information regarding this matter.

The recommended time for exercising your core muscles varies from one trainer to the other. Some of them may suggest you opt for an early morning routine. On the other hand, many trainers also give the advice of working out in the afternoon. So, it's entirely up to you as to which time will be suitable for you as per your lifestyle. But before you select a time, it is better to know the slight differences between the morning and afternoon workout routine.

Benefits of Exercising in the Morning

If you opt for this time of the day, then, first of all, it will turn out to be a consistent habit of yours. Getting up early morning and then tying up the laces of your sneakers help in building a consistent routine. The next advantage of doing core exercises early in the morning is that it will lessen your hunger. By practicing a morning exercise routine regularly, you will start observing that your rate of feeling hungry will gradually decrease. If you feel less hungry, the tendency to munch something or the other all throughout the day will also reduce to a certain extent. Those of you who are willing to burn extra fat or shed extra pounds by controlling your food habits may do the core exercises in the morning time. It will be easier for you to check your body weight. An adequate amount of sleep is necessary for people of almost all age groups. Exercising your core early in the morning before going out for work will assist you in falling asleep super quickly during nighttime. You will also be able to get sound sleep for nearly 7 to 8 hours.

Benefits of Exercising in the Afternoon

The level of stress hormone named cortisol is higher during the morning and starts reducing as the day passes. On the contrary, the production level of another hormone meant for muscle growth; testosterone, is higher in the afternoon time. This leads to a balance in the level of hormones. Thus, exercising your core muscles during this time of the day will become beneficial. Now, let's look forward to the next benefit of practicing core exercises in the afternoon. Just after we wake up in the morning, the muscles of every corner of our body remain stiff as the body takes a little time to wake up. Whereas if you exercise in the afternoon, your body will already become warmed up as you are completely awake by then. Your muscles will also not stay stiff and rather exhibit usual movements.

A maximum number of trainers agree on the common fact that night is not the best time for doing any sort of workout. By doing so, it may disrupt the internal clock or circadian rhythm of your body. Moreover, exercise has the potential to trigger your nervous system. Thus, if you practice exercise during nighttime, you may find it difficult to fall as well as stay asleep for a long time. No matter which time of the day you choose for exercising your core, the fact which is more important is trying your best to exercise steadily at your chosen time each day. You need to make daily appointments with yourself and, most importantly, take a vow to strengthen your core muscles through proper training. By doing so, you will be able to enjoy lifetime benefits.

Now that you have a brief idea regarding the time to exercise your core take a leap to the next part, where you will get certain information about the place for doing workouts. You will come across a variety of options while deciding the place to exercise. Whether you want to practice core exercises in public or private, it all depends on your financial condition, your comfort level, and your personal preference. A few options of where you can perform core workouts include:

- Gyms are excellent places for performing exercises, be it a renowned gym franchise or a local gym owned by any individual. It is true that you need to pay a certain amount of money on a monthly basis to get trained in a gym. But you will get various facilities such as various cardio equipment, free weights, exercise classes, weight machines, etc. Another benefit of using a gym is that you will stay in touch with an experienced trainer. If you wish to receive intensive guidance from a trainer to get guidance vis exercise routines, you just need to pay an additional wage. Besides strengthening your core muscles, you will also be able to connect and communicate with a lot of people in the gym. Thus, you will find it to be an all-over, fun-filled social experience.

- Another great option for those of you who are willing to choose a private space for doing core exercises is your home. If you have a vacant space inside your garage, a spare room, or any spot in your backyard, you may simply choose any of such spaces for exercising comfortably in the warmth of your home. One of the biggest advantages of exercising in your home is privacy and the convenience of not going to any other place just to maintain body fitness. Moreover, you will be able to perform workouts at your home even when you grow older. The best part of opting for this place is that it's free. No matter how long you practice or which corner you select, it's just free, free, and free! Unlike the gym, there is no specific time to exercise at home. If someday you feel like staying asleep for a longer time, you need not worry, as you will be able to perform workouts at any suitable time. It will not depend on the open hours of someone else.

- If you are looking for an open public space, then parks

full of greenery or some open fields will prove to be good options. Not only will you get to inhale the fresh air, but also enjoy the lush green color of mother nature. Such places are also cost-effective as there is no necessity to pay any charges for exercising in the open. It will also give you an opportunity to make friends with the other visitors and enjoy regular conversations with them. You will also feel the urge to visit your friends and thus never miss the chance to perform core exercises.

Thus, it's time for you to choose when and where to exercise your core. Keep reading for a lot more detailed information about certain myths and mistakes related to exercise, which almost all seniors must avoid for better body movement.

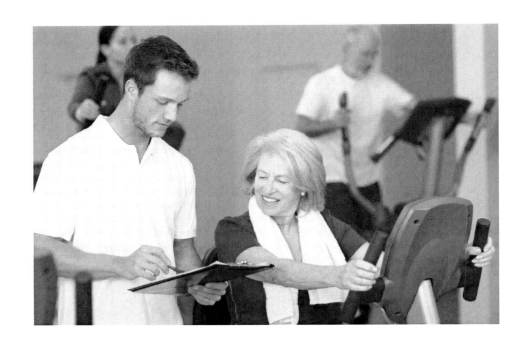

CHAPTER 5: MISTAKES AND MYTHS OF EXERCISE THAT SENIORS MUST AVOID

Staying fit is timeless. It creates a great difference in the way you move and feel. Fitness is also helpful in diminishing the numbers (such as blood pressure, cholesterol, or weight) that your physician keeps mentioning. Moreover, it also improves a person's mood. No matter what your age is, you win in every situation of your life when you are active both inside and outside. One of the amazing things one can do to support their health is entering a suitable exercise program. The need to stay involved in regular exercise increases as a person gets older. Not only will it let you experience enhanced ability and more energy to take part in regular activities, but it will also decrease the risk of the development of deep-rooted diseases, be it diabetes, heart disease, or dementia.

But the sad part is that a lot of people do exist who believe in certain myths related to exercise. Now, we will discuss a few common myths that senior citizens must avoid to enjoy life to the fullest.

Chiseled Abs Indicate Strong Core Muscles

This stands to be the first myth and also one of the most common ones. Are you a believer in this particular thought? If yes, then sorry to say that you will get exposed to the truth, and your belief will soon break. The aesthetic nature of your abs and the strength of your core muscles are two entirely different things. It does not mean that attaining six-pack abs is super easy. It requires both dedication and patience to wait for the desired outcome. If you possess a six-pack, then congratulations on attaining such an achievement. You might feel sad to know that your core muscles may lack stability and strength even if your muscles look well-defined and well-maintained. So, if you are truly willing to develop the power of your core, you must also rectify the imbalances of your back and chest.

Planks Give Six-Pack

First of all, you must know that planks are amazing for developing the strength of your core. But a lot of individuals hold a wrong belief that the lengthier a plank is held, the more advantageous it will be. Some are also there who think that doing a plank for five or six minutes will help them shed their abdominal muscles and give them a six-pack. You might feel disheartened to know this thought or myth is not true. What matters more is the quality of the plank and not the quantity. You will not be able to observe any positive results if you keep practicing an incorrect form. Furthermore, it is the usual tendency of a human body to get accustomed to repeated movements. That is the reason why one must perform various types of abdominal exercises. While planking, you may also try out variations such as keeping plates on your backside.

Old Persons Cannot Do Exercises

'I think I'm too aged for exercises, so it's better not to take the risk of giving it a try.' Numerous individuals who have started to grow old think that they are too old to practice regular core workouts. They think that age is an obstacle when the matter is about maintaining body fitness. It's high time that you need to throw away such myths from your mind. It is because staying inactive is a lot riskier and can also increase the speed of your aging process. Do you want to grow older faster or at a slow and regular pace? Most probably, your desire is to grow older at a slower pace, and then it is necessary to give up such thoughts and start becoming active. The chances of developing heart disease are double for those people who stay inactive and do not prefer movements. Such individuals also pay frequent visits to their physicians as well as consume more medications.

If you did not practice any sort of exercise in the long run, then it is better to start slowly with simple aerobic activities that are meant for elevating the heart rate, for example, swimming. Those who are willing to start a bit slower may opt for walking as a ten to fifteen minutes walk is an effective start. Is there any activity or workout you enjoyed during your younger days? If yes, you may look for ways of getting back to your old habits.

Exercise Makes the Heart Weaker

Do you think that your heart is not powerful enough to carry out regular core exercises? If you are willing to give an affirmative response to this question, then you need not worry, as you are not the only person holding such a thought. Your responsibility is to avoid this myth even if you are growing old and think and act differently. Suppose you start practicing exercises all of a sudden and give excessive effort on the very first day. No doubt you will feel exhausted, and your heart is beating faster than usual. It will force you to believe that your heart is weak and cannot withstand such hardships at this age. You need to start slowly and for a limited time period. No matter what your age is, it is always better to increase the time limit gradually. When practiced consistently, core exercises help strengthen your heart instead of putting it at any risk. There is no necessity to enroll your name for any marathon race. Staying physically active is also possible by taking a speedy walk. Such a walk is sufficient for controlling your cholesterol levels and blood circulation. Regular exercises are also beneficial in brightening your mood, which will keep your heart happy, even if you have crossed your sixties.

Core Exercises Help in Burning Belly Fat

Quite often, people get confused whenever their trainers suggest them to practice squats, burpees, or lunges to shed belly fat. The reason behind their confusion is the myth that keeps running in their minds regarding losing belly fat. A lot of individuals think that certain exercises, such as crunches, are far more effective as such workouts generate a sensation similar to burning all around the stomach area. That burning sensation is nothing other than the building up of lactic acid inside the muscle walls. It is not possible to reduce fat from a specific spot in your body. While performing workouts, your body sheds fat cells from every single corner.

Isolation Exercise Is the Most Effective Way to Develop Core Strength

The belief that the core muscles comprise only abdominal muscles has actually given rise to another misconception. Many people think that various forms of isolation exercises, such as Russian twists and crunches, are the most fruitful ways of building the strength of the core. Now, let's move ahead to know the truth so that it becomes easier for you to eliminate this myth completely from your mind. An isolation exercise is designed in such a manner that it enables supporting your spine along with making your regular movements easier even when your age increases by number. After all, the most efficient means of engaging your core muscles is via conscious breathing. By inhaling and exhaling intensely, your pelvis floor will get activated, and the intra-abdominal pressure will also get balanced.

Practicing Core Exercises Mean Getting Hurt

'I'm not in favor of performing core exercises at this age as I'll surely hurt myself.' It's time to stop thinking this way and give yourself some time to maintain your physical health. You will not at all hurt yourself if you do workouts within your personal limits and also if you know what and how to do. You must remember that the chances of getting injured will decrease only if you stay physically fit. To reduce the risk of getting hurt by falling down, you need to develop your body balance to a specific extent. Before starting any exercise program, you may also have a conversation with your physician. You will get an idea about the activities and exercises you may try and the ones you need to avoid.

Core Exercise Is Unaffordable

We get to hear a lot of people saying that they cannot afford such expensive workout programs. Many people stay away from core exercises as they believe in a myth like this. It is true that some individuals do pay to get a membership in any gym or purchase exercise equipment. But you need to spend a lot just for the sake of staying fit till the last days of your life. All you need to do is put on your sports shoes that are capable of providing good support to your feet and step out for a jog or walk. You may also spend an hour daily just gardening in your lawn or backyard. If someday you see that the weather is not good enough, utilize whatever is present at your home. You might get surprised to know that canned goods can also assist you in performing exercises. You may use canned goods to practice resistance training.

Besides this, utilizing your body weight for exercises such as pushups or planks also works wonders. Strolling up and down the staircase is also another form of simple workout. If, in any case, you are looking forward to making an investment in any machine, you may go for exercise equipment that is lightly used at yard sales in your locality. Those of you who are craving group fitness classes must not feel disappointed as there are various resources for staying fit. You will come across a few gyms that offer special discounts and health plans for senior citizens. Your task is to search for such gyms and enjoy staying flexible at an affordable rate. You may also take a look at the community resources. Certain local parks keep primary exercise equipment for seniors. You may also search for any local clubs where fitness classes are provided to all, especially elderly people, free of cost.

By now, you might have gained an idea about some of the myths that you must avoid and practice core exercises consistently as per your capability. So, the next part is knowing about the fitness or workout mistakes that seniors must avoid.

Skipping Warm-up

It is not at all a good idea to skip the warm-up. Many people, including seniors, tend to skip this part as they feel it to be unnecessary. Your overall body temperature increases and blood circulation also becomes normal after warming up your body. It is all about preparing the body for the forthcoming workout. Warming yourself up just before doing core exercises becomes more essential as a person starts aging. It is because aged people take more time than usual to overcome injuries. So, you need to make sure that you get prepared just before doing workouts. You just need a minimum time of five to ten minutes to warm yourself up. An excellent way of warming up is by performing the exercises that you have planned but at a slower pace.

Selecting the Incorrect Time for Stretching

Most individuals, including active senior citizens, usually perform static stretching before their workout. Sorry to say, but this is one of the most common mistakes that you need to avoid to improve your physical fitness. There is no wrong in doing static stretches, but choosing the wrong time is not appreciated at all. If you plan to practice static stretches, doing it after you finish your workout will give you a better outcome. The reason behind selecting the time just after workouts is because, at that moment, your muscles and joints will remain warm and thus more pliable. If your plan is to do a bit of stretching before workouts, then you may go for dynamic stretching. This form of stretching involves a variety of movements – such as alternative overhead reaches or walking lunges. If you use dynamic stretching as a part of warming up your body, it will assist you in gaining mobility as well as awakening your muscles before exercise.

Skipping Your Cooldown

The importance of cooling your body is almost similar to warming up. After you are done with your exercise, all the blood vessels become enlarged, your heart rate gets elevated, and the overall temperature of the body increases. If you cease the activities all of a sudden and do not allow yourself to cool down, chances are there that you may undergo poor blood pooling. In such a situation, you may feel dizzy or feel like losing consciousness. Now, this is when cooling down is necessary. Many people tend to skip this part to save time, but the result can be terrible. Cooldown enables you to slow your heart and breathing rate. Besides this, cooling down is one of the finest moments of your workout schedule, as it is meant for stretching and taking time to reflect on your exercise.

To enjoy the best results, you need to allow a minimum time of five to ten minutes to cool down your body. Instead of skipping this part, try out something that is light. For example, after the completion of jogging, an excellent cooldown will be to go for a short walk. One more means of cooling down is practicing some stretching, as it is helpful in calming and centering yourself.

Workout Forms Are Incorrect

Following good and proper forms of workout is not only applicable for young individuals but also for elder ones. Improper workout forms may build up or emphasize inferior movement patterns. If you go on performing exercises with incorrect form, then over time, it may lead to severe injury. Moreover, poor forms are also responsible for making your exercise routine less effective. Incorrect form means you are not targeting those muscles you are willing to engage in at the time of workouts. Usually, people practice incorrect forms as most of them do not receive the proper guidance from an expert. For improving your form, the best option is to seek the assistance of a professional trainer or train with your friend. If you do not have a workout companion, you may stand in front of your bedroom mirror and perform your exercises. It will assist you in checking whether you are utilizing the correct form and also let you engage the appropriate muscles throughout every move.

Neglecting Strength Training

Just like warming up and cooling your body, strength training is essential. It is required for developing strong muscles and also for retaining muscle tone. Weight lifting and resistance exercises enhance elasticity and strength and build powerful connective tissues. Many individuals make the mistake of skipping this part of strength training as most of them do not know its importance. If you follow strength training regularly, you will be able to do your daily activities with a lot more ease and comfort. It even enables increasing your metabolism; thus, it is one of the most effective ways to get rid of excessive body fat. Some people have a misconception that resistance training means lifting up weights. But the truth is something different. Body weight maintaining exercises such as push-ups, lunges, and activities including resistance bands are all helpful in building strong muscles.

Focusing particularly on Cardio

It is true that cardio is excellent for improving the health of your heart, amongst many other benefits. Thus, you may incorporate cardio into your workout or fitness routine. But, a lot of people keep their focus mainly on cardio, and this is indeed one of the most common workout mistakes that seniors need to avoid. Being an older adult, you must try to stay away from this mistake. Resistance and strength training can enhance a person's bone density and improve overall mobility by preventing Osteoporosis. You must make sure that you start lightly and then elevate your core strength over time.

Ignoring Nagging Injuries and Muscle Imbalances

Almost all of you might have noticed that the body's resistance level starts decreasing with age until and unless you move with deep intention. This type of muscle imbalance is more frequent among senior citizens. Elders suffer from muscle imbalances because of years of nagging injuries and poor posture. But the sad part and the worst mistake is ignoring such imbalances. A person is forced to depend on only one portion of their body just for the sake of muscle imbalance. Muscle imbalances also restrict an individual from using those muscles that are required for movement due to a lack of strength and mobility. So, you must not make the mistake of ignoring this sort of imbalance and thinking of ideas to correct them. Correcting imbalances is equally important as following perfect exercise forms.

Now that you are a bit aware of the mistakes seniors must avoid while exercising, it is better to avoid them to stay consistent and safe. *Let's move to the next part!*

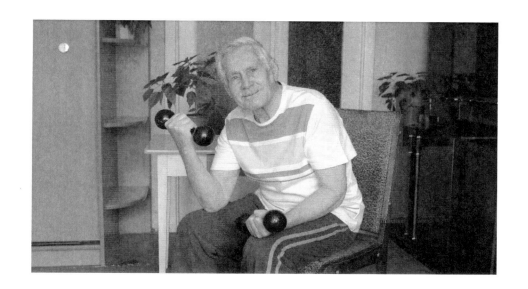

CHAPTER 6: SEATED CORE EXERCISES FOR SENIORS

A person who is sincere about fitness will definitely realize that regular physical activity is not only about losing weight. Exercise has a lot more to offer. Building your core strength is considered to be a lot more fruitful. It will indeed make your everyday movements such as running, walking, jumping, pushing, pulling, twisting, and bending much easier. Staying fit even as you grow older will let you be quicker and feel lighter on your feet. When you start working on your core, you indirectly begin to strengthen your whole body. However, a maximum number of individuals only seem to know such facts in theory. Usually, they fail to understand what is the exact matter to develop your core muscles. This chapter will tell you that it is possible to strengthen your core even while sitting.

To practice core exercises while you are sitting, you must choose modified workouts that emphasize holding postures, bracing your muscles, working against gravity, etc. You might be surprised to know that it is possible to strengthen your lower back, abs, obliques, and hips just by sitting down on a chair. Here are a few seated core exercises that might help people of almost all ages, especially seniors.

Forward Roll-Ups (Seated)

Are you willing to develop your functional core strength? If yes, seated forward roll-ups will work wonders. The muscle groups that are targeted for doing this workout are transverse abdominis and rectus abdominis. So, let's get started to know more about the steps on how to carry out this core exercise.

1. At first, you need to sit comfortably on a chair by keeping both your legs in an extended position. While extending your legs, you must be careful about putting your heels in contact with the floor. Let your feet stay flexed, pointing toward your face. Once you are done with this, stretch your arms in the forward direction. You are supposed to maintain a perfectly upright posture. Do not lean back or slouch.

2. After that, you need to curl your chin by bringing it towards your chest. Exhale while you roll your torso upwards and keep your abs engaged as well as your legs straight. Reach downwards in the direction of your toes.

3. As soon as you notice that you are finding it difficult to reach down further, start inhaling and rolling back towards your initial or starting position. You must not reach the starting point all at once; instead, do it slowly, such as a vertebra at one time.

4. Repeat the steps by moving slowly. It would be better if you avoid utilizing momentum and try using your abdominals for lifting and reaching down.

Seated Deadbug (Only Arms)

An effective and safe means of stabilizing and strengthening your core muscles is by following the seated deadbug exercise. It is helpful in developing your posture as well as assisting in giving you relief and preventing lower back pain. Most importantly, older adults will find it more beneficial as this exercise improves coordination and balance.

1. First of all, you are supposed to practice breathing techniques. For that, remain seated, maintaining a proper posture. Breathe deeply using your nose and not your mouth. While doing so, your belly and then your chest must expand.

2. After inhalation, the next step is to practice abdominal bracing. This term might be new to a lot of you. Abdominal bracing means flexing your abdominals hard. You need to hold this particular position.

3. Raise both your hands very slowly and keep them in such a position as if you are grasping a ball in front of your chest. Your hands are supposed to be in a parallel position with your face.

4. Raise an arm on top of your head by keeping your abdominals braced.

5. The next step is to lower that arm slowly and repeat the same with the other arm. If you are willing to modify this exercise by making it a bit more complicated, you may lift your opposite leg slightly from the ground simultaneously.

Side Bends (Seated)

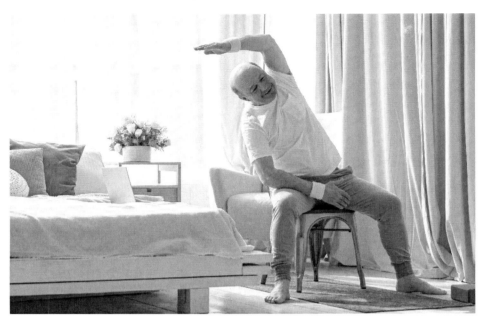

Are you looking for a core exercise that will enable you to relieve stress and relax your mind? You may go for a seated side bend if that is the case. This soothing exercise stretches the shoulders, neck, intercostals, obliques, triceps, and back. Apart from this, it even helps improve posture. Here are steps to perform this exercise:

1. For this, you need to sit on a chair by bending your knees and letting your feet touch the ground. Your next task is bending and bringing your right hand towards the right part of your head. While holding this posture, let your left arm hang by your side. Do not lean back and maintain an erect posture.

2. Now it's time to inhale. While exhaling, gently bend your waist to lower your left arm. Let it go towards the ground. You are supposed to open up your chest by pulling the right elbow backward. As you draw, you will feel that the right side of your body is stretching.

3. After that, you need to breathe in to come back to the

starting posture. Repeat.

Russian Twists (Seated)

One of the most effective means of building up your shoulders and core is practicing Russian twists regularly. It is beneficial in toning both your core muscles and shoulders. This exercise is quite popular among athletes as it includes rotational movement. Many of you might find the movements of this workout to be simple, but in reality, it requires immense support and strength. Let's look at the steps for performing the seated Russian twist.

1. Sit straight on a chair. Don't allow your back to bend.

2. The next step is bending your knees at a right angle. If you want it to be more advanced, lift your feet one inch off the floor.

3. Use your hands to make a tight fist, and hold the fist just in front.

4. After that, tighten your core muscles. Bring your clasped hands from one side to the other. Follow your moving hands with your eyes and head. If the chair on which you are sitting has arms, your aim must be to touch each side.

5. Sit in an upright posture, and breathe from beginning to end. You must practice to brace your abdominals during every single repetition. (You may do a total number of 20 repetitions, 10 per side. Take a break of 45 seconds and then go for two more sets.)

Seated Leg Tap

Such an exercise is helpful in toning your entire body, especially your core. A seated leg tap helps in enhancing the strength of your lower body and even elevates your heart rate. It is beneficial for senior people as it enables them to improve flexibility. The steps are here for you:

1. Sit on a strong chair by bending your knees to perform this core exercise. Keep your feet on the floor in a flat position. You need to maintain an upright position and remember not to lean back or slouch.

2. Use both your hands to hold the bottom portion of the seat to get enough support. After this, engage your abs and try extending the legs on the front side. Use both your feet to tap the ground.

3. Pull both your legs underneath the chair to reset your position. Let your feet rest on the ground. Once you are prepared, repeat the steps.

Bend Over Reverse Fly

The benefits of reverse fly exercise are numerous, so it is treated as one of the most effective ways to strengthen your core muscles. It is helpful in making your shoulders strong, which will prevent you from getting injured while performing various other moves. This workout is known to support shoulder girdle as well as improve posture to a great extent. To perform bend over the reverse fly, you need to follow the following steps:

1. You first need to take a chair and sit on its edge carefully. Before you start with the workout, take one huge diaphragmatic breath. Let your spine stay in a neutral position and breathe in through your nose. While exhaling, be attentive about bracing your abdominals.

2. Your next task is to maintain this exact pressure in the core muscles and then lean slightly in the forward direction. While leaning forward, you are supposed to engage your back. Now, it's time to create a proud chest position.

3. You must start by keeping your arms in front of your

body and allowing the palms to face each other.

4. Your responsibility is to maintain the proud chest or tight back position. After that, lift your arms straight to the side portion of your body so that you look similar to the English alphabet 'T.' You are to hold this posture for a second.

5. Slowly, come back to the beginning position. The slower you return, the better the outcome will be. (Experts suggest practicing three sets of a total number of ten to fifteen repetitions.)

Knee Tucks or Single Leg Lift

Do you desire to lose weight from your lower abdomen and legs? If you have an affirmative response, a single leg lift will suit you. Besides losing excessive weight, this particular core exercise is beneficial in toning and strengthening your leg and abdominal muscles. It will even assist you in making your calf muscles, glutes, and hamstrings strong. Knee tucks will enable you to enhance your endurance and strength in a very short time span. It also helps in flattening your belly as well as provide some intense and quick cardio benefits. Well, the steps are pretty simple. Have a look!

1. At first, you need to sit either on edge or middle of a chair. As you are done with the sitting part, maintain a good posture as well as a neutral spine.

2. After that, you are supposed to keep both your hands near your glutes or thighs. Grip the chair firmly.

3. Bend your right leg and raise it as much high as possible. Your aim must be to lift your bent leg above the height of your hip. Hold this posture for a second when your leg is at the topmost position.

4. After returning your first leg to the initial position, you

need to do the same with the other leg. If ever you wish to make this exercise more advanced, you must make an attempt to keep both your legs straight.

Half Roll-Back (Seated)

Half-roll back is better known for training the transverse abdominis, the rectus abdominis, and the lower and upper abdominals. Thus, incorporating this core exercise into your weekly routine will be a brilliant move. It is an excellent way to warm your body gently as well as prepare it for more. So, let's learn the steps for practicing this workout.

1. Take a chair and sit by keeping your feet flat and knees bent. Now, raise both your arms so as to make a circle in front of your chest. While doing this, you must not lean back or bend. It is mandatory to keep an erect posture.

2. Let your arms remain in that circle posture, and touch the floor with your feet. Start rounding your back. While doing this, you must remember to scoop your abdominals.

3. When you observe that you are unable to move further, start rolling your back slowly to go to the initial position. Don't forget to engage your abdominals.

Tummy Twist

This exercise is not only meant for your entire core but also for stretching your spine. You may perform this workout with the help of one medicine ball. In case you do not get such a ball, you may use any similar object. Here are the steps:

1. At first, you need to hold the medicine ball.

2. Make yourself comfortable by sitting on the edge of a chair. By sitting on the edge, you will get extra space. Tighten both your lumbar and abdominals and stick

your chest in the outward direction. You must place both your hands in the front of your body and bend your elbows to hold the medicine ball.

3. After that, your next task is to raise the ball a few inches above your lap and start rotating the upper part of your body in the right direction. While you rotate your body, be careful about keeping that ball in the front.

4. Now, it's time to rotate towards the left, but before that, you need to turn your body to the middle. A set will complete after returning to the middle portion. Every set includes a full rotation.

It is time-consuming to build up a strong core. But once you go with the flow, it will provide you stability and balance for doing all your regular activities with ease. The time required to strengthen your core is dependent on the present condition and strength of your core muscles. You must not rush and be impatient. Different core strengthening workouts must be followed to ensure that every inch of the midsection is hit properly. Your age, past injuries, or mobility restrictions must not stop you from including the above-mentioned seated core workouts in your daily routine. Just remain seated; it's just that simple. Turn the page as the time has come to strengthen your core muscles by using a mat.

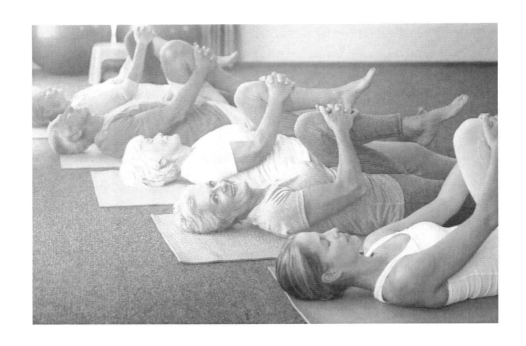

CHAPTER 7: CORE EXERCISES USING ONLY YOUR MAT

People start facing a lot of challenges with age, such as decreased bone density and strength, muscle weakness, etc. All such obstacles affect balance, gait, and coordination. To get rid of such difficulties, all you need to do is aim to strengthen your muscles. By doing so, you will be able to regain your bone and muscle strength, mobility rate, flexibility, fitness, and balance. This chapter will help you learn the procedure of performing a few core exercises; for that, all you require is an exercise mat. Have a look at the details!

Superman

Is superman your favorite fictional character? If yes, then quickly bring your mat for performing a core exercise having the same name. This workout helps to strengthen your glute muscles and upper and lower back. Strengthening all these muscles will enable you to practice any sort of movement that requires sitting or bending over. Have a look at the steps that are mentioned below for your convenience.

1. First of all, take a mat and use it for cushioning. Begin the workout by lying on the mat with your face facing downwards.

2. Your arms must be stretched in the front direction. Start lifting an arm, along with the opposite leg and your head. Lift all the mentioned body parts almost two inches from the mat.

3. Be sure not to forget to squeeze the glutes, as it will help you remove some pressure from the lower back side. You must also pretend to have one marble in the belly button. Pretend to squeeze that marble hard too.

4. Once you are done doing all these steps, lower your raised body parts to repeat the same steps using the opposite side. It is better to do four to five repetitions on every single side. (If you find these steps to be a bit difficult for you, you may try to maintain the posture by lifting only your arms. Once you build up the necessary strength, try lifting your legs.)

Bird Dog

This is one of the simplest core exercises that help improve stability and provides relief from lower back pain. It even encourages to maintain a neutral spine. The posture of this workout uses the entire body and targets as well as strengthens the hips, back, and core muscles. Besides this, bird dog exercise is also beneficial in promoting perfect body posture and also enhances the range of motion. Older adults who are willing to develop spinal stability may go for this particular workout and observe the positive outcome. Here are the steps that will help you to perform this exercise.

1. Get on the limbs on your mat. After getting down on all fours, engage all your core muscles and try keeping your neck, head, and spine in one line.

2. Now, lift the left leg upwards and allow it to extend behind you.

3. After that, raise your opposite hand, i.e., the right hand, off the mat and stretch it in the front.

4. Once you attain this posture, hold it for five to ten seconds.

5. Your next task is to return to the initial position.

6. Now, raise the right leg from the mat and spread it just behind you.

7. Lift the left hand and let it stretch in your front.

8. Again, you are supposed to hold this pose for the time mentioned above.

9. Return to the beginning position and repeat this entire set thrice.

Forearm Plank

If you can do this exercise in the correct procedure, you may find it a bit tough. Even though it's difficult, you will feel excited after knowing its benefits. It helps strengthen your legs, core muscles, and abdominals. Moreover, this workout is also excellent for extending the arches of both your calves and feet, hamstrings, and shoulders. Most importantly, the forearm plank lets an individual work on their core without any risk of getting a back injury. Thus, elders must not feel scared to try this workout. Here are the ways to practice this exercise:

1. Lie down on a mat with your face facing downwards. Let your forearms rest on the mat. The position of your elbows has to be underneath your shoulders and keep both your elbows wide apart.

2. Get prepared by engaging your core. Apply force with the help of your forearms to lift your body off the mat. You will get the required support from your toes and forearms.

3. Your entire body, i.e., starting from your head towards your feet, must remain in one straight line. After that, you are to pull the navel into the spine as well as squeeze the glutes. By doing so, your hips won't drop down towards the mat.

4. It is necessary to hold this position for a minimum time span of thirty seconds or a minute. (If you observe that you cannot maintain the straight line between your hips and shoulders, you may drop your knees. You may also do the same if you feel a slight pressure in the lower back portion of your body.)

Pilates Hundred

Now, this is a great exercise for warming up your abdominal muscles. It is even helpful in oxygenating your body. Pilates hundred enhances blood circulation, develops stability, endurance, and strength, and also builds up the abdominal muscles. To do this exercise, you have to coordinate your body movements with your breathing. Look at the steps:

1. Start this workout by lying down on your back and keeping both legs in a tabletop position, which means your knees and hips will be at right angles. The next step

is to engage your abdominals to give a round shape to the lower portion of your spine while staying in touch with the mat. Make sure that you are not just working on the upper layer of your abs.

2. After that, breathe out and raise the upper back from the mat. Keep lifting until your shoulder blades leave the floor. Now, you have to unfold your legs by maintaining an angle of 45-degree. While straightening your legs, you must be careful about keeping your lower back connected to the mat. Try reaching towards your feet with the help of your arms. The gap between the floor and your arms must be about two inches.

3. Your next task is to straighten your elbows to pump your arms in an upward and downward motion. Inhale and then exhale for five arm pumps each. That will complete a cycle or set. You need to repeat this set nine more times, which will sum up to a total of a hundred pumps.

4. You must not forget to keep the upper portion of your body stable while you pump your arms.

Bridge

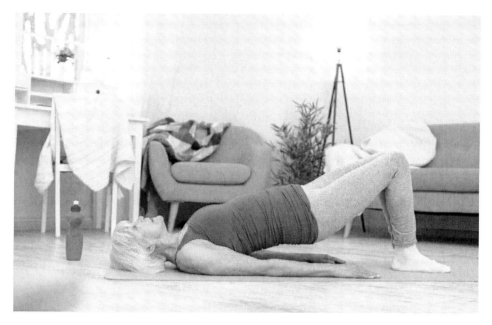

The bridge exercise is an excellent way to strengthen your posterior chain, which is an essential part of your core, including the hips, glutes, abdominals, and lower back. By practicing this core exercise, you will be able to keep your disks and spine in perfect alignment. This, in turn, will let you move comfortably and freely without any sort of pain. Here's how to do bridge:

1. Start this exercise by lying down on a mat with your face facing the upward direction. Bend your legs at a right angle to the mat.

2. After this, you need to engage your core and glutes and try pushing your hips upward.

3. Hold this posture for one beat, then gently lower your body parts. Touch the floor.

4. Repeat the steps mentioned above for five to ten reps, and breathe in between.

Cat Cow

The cat cow pose is good for boosting the flexibility of your shoulder, spine, and neck. The movement included in this exercise helps to extend the muscles of your back, abdomen, chest, and hips. Moreover, the stretch involved in this workout is helpful in releasing the tension of your upper back and neck as well as calming your mind. It is even known for warming up your body. You will be able to open up your chest and encourage your breath to become intense and slow. Besides all these, the cat cow exercise develops your body balance and posture. If practiced regularly, this workout will enable to ward off back pain. Now, let's go through the steps involved in this core exercise:

1. Start by keeping your knees and hands in a table pose. Make sure that your spine is in the neutral position. To prepare for the cow pose, you need to inhale and raise your sit bones in an upward direction, let your belly sink, and push your chest forward.

2. After that, lift your head and allow your shoulders to relax. Your gaze must be straight ahead.

3. Now, while exhaling, you will enter into the cat pose, and you need to round your spine in the exterior portion. Ensure you tuck your tailbone inside and extend the pubic bone in the front.

4. Once you are done with all these steps, loosen your head and let it move towards the mat. Do not let your chin move towards your chest forcefully. At this stage, the most crucial part is to relax.

One Leg Crunch

One leg or single leg crunch, as you may call it, is one of the most common core exercises that is performed using an exercise mat. The movement involved in this workout is effective for both the upper and lower abdominal muscles. It even targets your obliques and hip flexors. This one-leg crunch is beneficial for enhancing your flexibility, core strength, and leg stretch. You may come across different variations of leg crunches. Here are specific instructions that will help you quickly learn the single leg crunch.

1. In the beginning, you have to lie down on your exercise mat. Bend both your knees after lying and keep your hands under your head.

2. The next step that you need to follow is raising your head, shoulders, and neck off the mat. Lift all these parts by shrinking your abdominals. Simultaneously, lift up a bent knee until you observe that the thigh is in a perpendicular position to the mat.

3. After that, start lowering the upper back of your body. While doing so, remember to stretch your leg. Repeat the set with the other leg.

T-Cross Sit-up

You will indeed be contented to know that this exercise works on all your abdominal muscles. The targets of this workout are oblique muscles and rectus abdominis. Those of you who are looking for a core exercise to lose fat may include this in your body fitness routine. It is even helpful in tightening your body because it deeply affects your obliques. Let's learn the steps quickly for staying fit and flexible even when you start aging!

1. To begin with, lie down on a mat. Open up both your arms widely on both sides. This will give your body the posture of the letter T.

2. Once you are comfortable, get up and sit and, at the same time, raise the right leg. Now, you need to twist a bit so that you can touch your right toes with the left hand. After reaching your toes, roll back your body slowly in the initial position. Relax for one or two seconds and repeat the same on the opposite side. This will complete one set.

Windshield Wiper

It is even known as a modified windshield wiper or lying windshield wiper. The target of this particular bodyweight exercise is your core muscles. This workout involving your entire body is known to activate various muscle groups. Some of the basic muscles targeted while performing this workout are obliques, rectus abdominis, hip flexors, erector spinae, etc. If you are able to do the windshield wiper exercise properly, it will resemble a car's wiper. It develops muscle strength, provides improved sleep quality, prevents back pain, and boosts coordination and balance. This core exercise even aids in losing weight. If you perform this workout regularly, it will help release certain feel-good hormones, which are helpful in improving your mood. Are you excited to know the steps that are involved in the lying windshield wiper exercise? If yes, then the steps are here only for you.

1. Lie down comfortably on your mat. Stretch out both your arms and keep them at right angles from the shoulders. Push your arms and palms firmly into the floor just for the sake of stabilizing your spine and shoulders.

2. Now, lift up your legs and then bend both knees by making an angle of 90 degrees. The posture should be as if you are seated on a chair.

3. In a very controlled and slow motion, let down your feet to a side. Next, you need to drag the belly button towards your spine. Lifting your spine slightly when you start turning your body would be best. But you must also try keeping your spine pressed into the mat as much and as long as possible.

4. Once you are done with all these steps, your next task is lifting your legs to the initial position by engaging your abs.

5. Repeat all the steps by pushing down the opposite side. This will complete one set.

You may consult your physician before starting the exercises if you want. Many seniors keep looking for activities that can be done in a standing position. So, the next chapter is for you all who are eagerly waiting for standing core exercises.

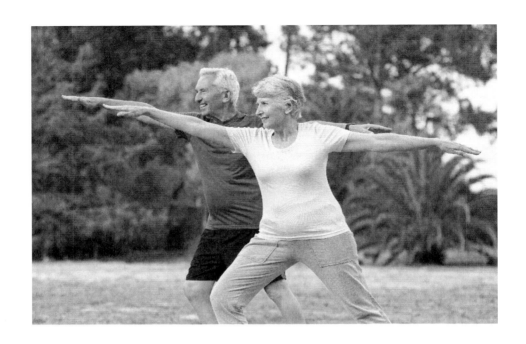

CHAPTER 8: STANDING CORE EXERCISES FOR SENIORS

By now, all of you are well aware of the importance of a strong core. From walking to lifting weights or doing regular activities, having stable and active core muscles help make a huge difference. In the previous chapters, you encountered a few core exercises that can be practiced by sitting or using an exercise mat. Here you will get information about standing core exercises that might help seniors to activate their core muscles. Core exercises that can be practiced by simply standing help strengthen your deeper core muscles as well as your obliques. Such exercises are an efficient tool for defining and strengthening your abdominal muscles. The various forms of standing core exercises are excellent for building up and strengthening the muscles from your hips to your back.

Now it's time to learn some of the standing core exercises in detail. *Have a look!*

Woodchop

This powerful exercise has a lot of advantages. People who are unable to lie down to work on their core may try the woodchop exercise as it is an efficient means to work their trunk muscles. It even improves the strength of the muscles present in your hips and shoulders. Besides your hip and trunk muscles, your calf and thigh muscles are also involved in this exercise. This core strengthening exercise is also helpful in enhancing your posture and balance as well as toughening your lower and upper body. While doing this movement, you need to maintain the stability of your trunk. Usually, people tend to bend or flex their spine in the forward direction during the woodchop exercise. If such a situation, then your spine may get stressed. But you need not worry as you may try using lighter weights. Now, let's go through the steps:

1. At first, you are supposed to stand upright and maintain a gap in between your feet (shoulder-width). Take a dumbbell and hold it carefully using both hands.

2. Then, start rotating your torso towards the right side. As you turn, lift the dumbbell till you make it reach over your right shoulder.

3. Let down your body by bending your knees while twisting the torso to the opposite side. At the same time, carry your dumbbell in a diagonal position across your body. Make sure that the dumbbell is near your left hip.

4. Repeat all the steps mentioned earlier and follow the same process by switching sides. (You will enjoy better outcomes if you let your knees and feet point in a similar

direction and also straighten your arms. While twisting your torso, you must not forget to breathe out and engage the core muscles.)

Oblique Bend (Standing)

The main target of the oblique standing bend is the internal and external obliques. It even makes the side abdominal wall strong. If you are willing to try some exercise that will enable you to tighten your core, sculpt your waist, and develop your stability and posture, you may surely go for this one. By practicing this workout regularly, the pressure that you feel on your lower back while doing daily activities like lifting heavy things will start reducing. So, here are the steps:

1. In the beginning, you are to stand straight. Check that your feet are wide apart from each other, for example, hip-width. Your hands must be at the back of your head, and keep your elbows wide.

2. Once you are ready with the above-mentioned posture, raise and bring the right knee towards the right elbow. You will be able to do so only if you curve your torso over your right side. That is one set. You need to do a total number of ten such sets. After that, your task is to switch sides and repeat the same process.

Warrior Balance

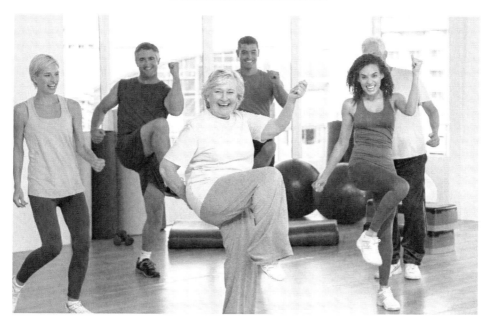

The first and foremost advantage of warrior balance exercise is that it enables you to strengthen your legs, build up core strength, and improve balance. Besides tightening your legs and standing ankle, this balancing exercise is also known for toning your abdomen as well as boosting posture. By performing this workout properly, you will notice that your level of stamina for doing your daily chores has also elevated a lot more than before. Let's jump in to know the steps:

1. Stand! Use your right foot for standing. As you observe that you are able to maintain proper balance while standing on one foot, raise your left knee to the height of your hip. You have to lift your knee in the front part of the body.

2. Next, you need to make your torso reach forward and then stretch your left leg in the backward direction. When your torso attains a parallel position with the ground or mat, your task is to bend the leg on which you are standing slightly. You may stretch both arms over your head to help your body maintain the necessary

balance.

3. Just pause for a fraction of a second, and reverse all the movements. That will make one complete set, and it would be better if you are able to complete ten such repetitions. After that, switch the sides and continue the same with the opposite side.

Standing March and Twist

Marching movements help in creating stability on either side of your body, i.e., glutes and hip flexors. Now, if you include twists along with marching, it will let you develop the required balance while enhancing the stability of your core muscles. The muscles that can be activated with the help of twists include quadratus lumborum, transverse and rectus abdominis, external and internal obliques, spinal erectors, etc. You won't need any equipment to do this exercise. You need to follow the instructions mentioned below:

1. To perform the standing march along twist, stand in an erect position by keeping your feet wide apart. Touch the back side of your head lightly with your fingertips. Open up your elbows to both sides. You must not pull or put pressure on your head.

2. Bring your left elbow towards your right knee and twist your body through the waist. After that, come back to the initial position. Repeat the same using the right elbow and left knee.

3. Continue alternating sides for a minute. (While lifting your knee, you must be careful to use your core muscles and not the quads. You must also squeeze your oblique muscles throughout the movement.

Standing Side Reach

Are you looking for an effective workout to awaken your core? If yes, then you are at present in the correct place. All you need to do is stretch your body by practicing side reaches. This exercise will strengthen and stretch your intercostal muscles, i.e., the muscles in between your ribs. Besides this, side-reach exercise will reduce back pain, improve your posture, and develop various motions. Seniors will find it to be more appealing when they get to know that this core exercise assists in enhancing blood flow. Steps on how to perform this exercise:

1. Stand by keeping a shoulder-width distance between your feet. Let your arms relax on both sides.

2. Once you are set with the initial posture, breathe in and drag your left arm on top of your head. At the same time, lean towards the right by extending the right side of your body.

3. After that, breathe out and come back to the starting position, i.e., the center.

4. Now, repeat the same steps using the other side of your body.

Deadlift Using Single Leg

Unilateral movements that include only one arm or leg; challenge your overall body balance and core. The single-leg deadlift is an effective and simple exercise for toning and strengthening your butt muscles. Most importantly, it is known for improving posture and balance and also developing muscle strength. If you incorporate this exercise into your regular workout routine, you will get to observe increased core stability after a few days. Willing to learn the steps for attaining a more stable core? Well, the steps are here for you:

1. At first, you have to stand and maintain a shoulder distance between your feet. Keep your arms by your side.

2. Now, start inhaling. Breathe out and start bending from

the waist. Your bending posture will be like this – the left leg has to be straight just behind you, along with your arms stretched on the front side of your body.

3. You must be careful about your hips not opening up. Let the hips be in a square posture with the floor. Slightly bend the right knee so that you can feel the floor beneath you.

4. You must take your extended leg back as far as possible until you are comfortable. The main aim of this exercise is to form one straight line starting from your fingers to your toes. After that, return to the starting position.

5. Repeat the steps of a single-leg deadlift using the right leg.

Triangle Pose

The triangle pose exercise is great for beginners and those who are a bit more advanced. It is not only simple but also quite effective in benefitting your mental and physical health. This exercise will activate your core, which in turn, will aid in stability and balance. Core activation also leads to stimulation of the digestive organs. Hence, your metabolism will also develop after you start performing this traditional exercise. This particular pose also can decrease stiffness in your back and spine, which results in improving flexibility. It even opens your shoulders and chest. The standing triangle posture targets your lower back, and it is the place where a maximum number of individuals bear their stress. Thus, it is helpful in releasing such tension, and the outcome is minimized anxiety along with a calm and strong emotional state. Here are the key steps that you need to follow while practicing this advantageous standing core exercise:

1. Your first task is positioning your body. For this, you have to stand by moving your feet a bit wider than your shoulder width. Stretch your arms with the palms

facing downward. Your arms must maintain a parallel position with the flow. Suppose you are willing, to begin with your right side, that the angle between your right foot and the floor must be a 90-degree. At the same time, the left foot must be at an angle of 45- degrees.

2. Once you are done with the above-mentioned position, your next task is to bend to your side. Inhale deeply and then exhale slowly while bending your body just from your hip joint. Keep the pressure of your entire body on your right leg, and then extend your body to a side. Do not scrunch your waist, and let the sides of the waist stay long. After that, you have to elongate the tailbone towards the back of your heel.

3. Well, the next step is reaching down using your arms. For this, you have to reach your right foot with the help of your right arm. Grip your ankle gently with the right hand. While reaching down, you are supposed to stretch the left arm in the upward direction simultaneously. Remember to point all the fingers of this hand towards the sky or ceiling. By doing so, you will be able to form a vertical and straight line with your shoulders and arms. (You must not bend your knees while reaching down, and try keeping your leg straight.)

4. Let your shoulders remain aligned. Move your head to look up at the ceiling. Hold this position for a few seconds, and then come back to the initial position. Repeat the same with your left leg. (While performing the triangle pose exercise, you must avoid curving your back or rounding up your spine.)

Hip Circles

Hip circles are one of the greatest and most progressive stretching exercises. It assists in loosening your hip muscles and lower back muscles. Strengthening your core muscles is another benefit of performing hip circles. If you perform this standing core exercise in the proper form, you will be able to trim your waist. Besides all these advantages, this workout helps relieve tension and stress and also develops your flexibility. Those who are willing to bring smooth movement to their hips may opt for hip circles. You will be able to enjoy a relaxed feeling after practicing this exercise. Steps for doing the hip circles exercise are mentioned below:

1. Stand on your feet with a gap of shoulder width. Put both your hands on the hips.

2. Fix your feet firmly on the floor. Start drawing a circle using your hips by moving it in a clockwise direction.

3. Enlarge the circle when you feel that your hips are getting looser.

4. Repeat the above-mentioned process, but this time, make your hips move in an anti-clockwise direction.

The moves mentioned in this chapter are the top exercises meant for individuals of all age groups, especially older adults. It will help if you keep a target of doing such core exercises regularly so that you can maintain healthy and strong core muscles. If, by chance, you experience any sort of sharp pain or discomfort during exercise, you must stop practicing immediately and consult with your physician for better guidance.

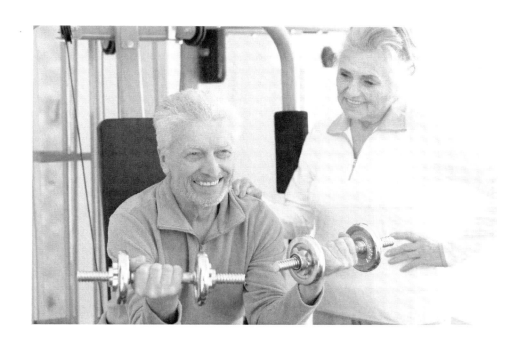

CHAPTER 9: CORE EXERCISES USING WEIGHTS

The muscle group that has the potential to break or create your fitness capabilities is nothing other than your core. The basis of stability and balance is a healthy and active core. It will also aid you in building up muscle mass efficiently. One of the finest ways to strengthen your core is by including weights, be it heavy or light. If you can build a stronger core with the help of weighted exercises, you will gain better balance, posture, muscle stability, and flexibility. Senior citizens might feel contented to know that improved flexibility is connected with fewer injuries and better overall performance.

Core exercises using weights might be a bit challenging, but their countless benefits will encourage you to proceed further. In this chapter, you will come across a few effective core exercises that will involve weights. *Hopefully, you will have a good read!*

Dumbbell Side Bend

If you involve this particular core exercise in your fitness or strength-gaining program, it is doubtless that you will enjoy several benefits. First of all, it helps improve core strength. As the target muscles of the dumbbell side bend are external and internal obliques, so it possesses the potential to build up the sides of a person's body. Moreover, your spinal and functional mobility will also get developed because of this core exercise using weights. With proper form and regular practice, dumbbell side bend helps strengthen your spine's lateral flexion. This exercise is easy enough to try at home. Want to know the process of performing such an advantageous exercise? Okay, the steps are here:

1. Stand erect by maintaining a gap of hip- or shoulder-width in between your feet. Take one dumbbell in your right hand and let your knees bend slightly. Your overall posture has to be tall, and a correct posture can be attained by maintaining an alignment between your hips and your shoulders. It is also necessary to keep your neck and head in a neutral position.

2. The next step is placing your left hand at your head's back. You must not pull your head in the front. During the movement, your chin needs to remain tucked. It must appear as if there is an egg underneath your chin, and you are holding it firmly. You need to distribute your body weight evenly and hold the floor tightly using your feet. A stable position can be created in this manner.

3. Next, you need to grip the dumbbell with the palms facing the forward direction. Keep your arm's length and let your elbow bend slightly. While you start to engage your core, it is necessary to pre-tension both your hips

and shoulders. Every single repetition must start from this position.

4. Bend the spine towards the right slowly and, in the meantime, keep the rest part of your body fixed or motionless. The dumbbell will move downwards as you bend to the right and stay just over your knee.

5. After that, squeeze your lateral core and left oblique muscles and start dragging your body towards the left.

6. You must squeeze the left oblique continuously until you observe that the upper portion of your body is bending slightly towards the left. The look will be almost similar to a side crunch. Pause, squeezing as you reach the end of this movement or as far as you feel comfortable.

7. Now straighten the spine slowly and continue the same set by switching sides. (You must not lean backward or forward while bending to the sides. Do it smoothly and slowly.)

Weighted Crunch

While talking about core exercises using weights, the weighted crunch will surely be there on the list. Whether you perform standing or seated weighted crunch, doing any variation will help in building a strong core. This, in turn, prevents injuries by stabilizing your back. Not only does this exercise develop your posture, but it also prevents stiffness and any sort of pain in the lower back. Your endurance level and muscle strength will enhance with the help of this exercise. It means you will become more active as well as gain a well-toned appearance. Moreover, weighted crunch also helps to develop bone density along with preventing certain degenerative conditions like osteoporosis. This core exercise using weights aids in elevating the heart rate, which in turn promotes fitness and wealth because of an improved cardiovascular system. Now that you are well aware of the benefits of the weighted crunch, it's time for you to know the steps to perform this workout in detail. Look ahead!

1. Lie down on your exercise mat with your face facing upwards, knees slightly bent, making a right angle, and feet touching the floor. While lying in this position, take hold of a dumbbell and try holding it to your chest as close as possible. Both your pelvis and spine have to be in a non-aligned position. You must also check that your ribs are down and the pelvis is slightly tucked.

2. Your core needs to be engaged properly. Your arms have to remain crossed while gripping the dumbbell. It is the beginning position.

3. After this, your next task is to start crunching. For this, you must lift your head and shoulders off the floor. It is also necessary to crunch your ribcage towards the pelvis. Just hold this posture for a short time span. Then lower your back slowly to return to the starting position.

4. You may repeat the steps as necessary. (Make sure not to jerk your body and let the movements be very slow.)

Reverse Dumbbell Chop

This weight-involved core exercise helps build up your core muscles' functional strength. A reverse dumbbell chop actually prepares your core so that it can stabilize your whole body in all possible directions. The muscles that are targeted in this exercise are the core, quads, and shoulders. If you are willing to make the exercise a bit easier, you may involve a lighter dumbbell. Bending your knees a little is also helpful in making the exercise easier. After regular practice, if you start feeling it's time to make it difficult, just do the opposite: practice with a heavyweight. So, go through the procedure so that you get to comprehend the exercise properly.

1. Use both your hands to grasp a dumbbell of your

preferred weight. While you hold the dumbbell, stand straight in such a manner so that there is a gap of hip width between your feet. After that, start rotating your torso towards the left side after bending your knees. Rotate in a way so that both your hands remain on the outer portion of the left thigh.

2. Now, you are to keep the arms straight and start swinging the weight slowly. The swinging needs to be done diagonally across the torso. Make sure that the dumbbell stays over the right shoulder while straightening your legs.

3. Next, you must reverse the steps to come back to the initial posture. That will complete one set, and you will get a good result if you practice doing ten such sets. Then, your task is to switch the sides and repeat the same steps and an equal number of repetitions.

Core Stabilizer

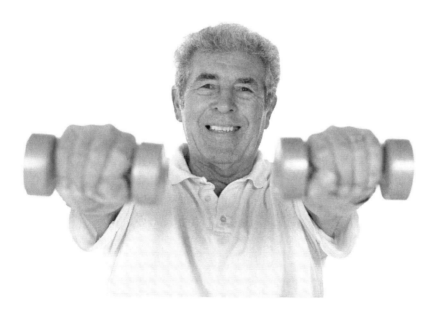

As the name suggests, the main aim of core stabilizer exercise is to strengthen your core muscles. Besides this, this particular core exercise also assists an individual in learning the various ways of using the internal muscles before any sort of movement. The major focus remains on enhancing the stability of the core. Here are the steps that one must follow while performing this workout.

1. First of all, concentrate and stand straight comfortably. While standing, keep your feet wide apart. Once you are done with this posture, take a dumbbell and hold it straight with your hands just on the front side of your chest.

2. Now, your next responsibility is to move the torso to some extent. After that, start rotating your arms slowly in the right direction. Rotate only as far as you feel comfortable.

3. Pause for only one second. After taking such a short break, rotate your hands in the reversed direction. This will complete one set. Do ten similar sets for outstanding outcomes. (You must hold the weight properly while you perform the rotating part.)

Knee Tuck Extension (Using Weight)

If you are looking for a workout that will assist you in improving your endurance level and core strength, and that too in a very short time span, you may try out knee tuck extension, including weight. Besides elevating the strength of your core, it is even helpful in toning and shaping your entire body. Older adults will find this exercise to be quite beneficial as they will get an opportunity to keep their bodies in shape, even after growing older. This exercise is effective in letting you control your movements. It emphasizes your hip flexors and abdominal muscles. The main muscles involved in this workout are the rectus and transverse abdominis, external and internal oblique muscles, and quadriceps. An amazing benefit of choosing this exercise is that it can be done anytime and anywhere. The steps are here for your convenience:

1. Maintain a shoulder-width gap between your feet and stand erect. Your next task is to bend your arms by holding one dumbbell with each hand. Keep the weights above your shoulders.

2. Now, bend the torso towards the right side and, at the same time, bring the right knee upwards. Your aim must be to touch your elbow to your knee. Make sure that the entire movement remains concentrated to a side.

3. Lastly, return to the starting posture. Repeat all the steps by involving the opposite side.

Overhead Circles

The subtle movements involved in overhead circles might appear to be easy, but once you engage it perfectly, your entire core will get fired up. This weight-involved exercise targets a person's shoulders and assists in toning as well as strengthening your core and upper body. Other than this, overhead circles are also helpful for developing the range of shoulder movements. This, in turn, decreases the chances of getting injured. Steps on how to perform overhead circles are here:

1. You may use a dumbbell or a medicine ball to do this workout. Stand with your feet wide apart, such as the width of your shoulder. Hold the dumbbell at the two ends and extend your arms just overhead.

2. Grip the floor firmly with your feet and also involve your core muscles to draw circles. Use your dumbbell to draw a circle over your head. While doing this, you are to rotate your torso for a smoother movement.

3. First, move clockwise as many number of times are

you wish to. After that, start doing the same in an anticlockwise direction. Yes, it's just that easy!

Thus, if you include weighted core exercises in your workout routine, it will surely assist you in reaching your desired fitness goals in the long run. But if you have any health issues, you may consult with your practitioner to receive better guidance on whether you should use weights to train your core or not. For the time being, let's move to the next interesting part.

CHAPTER 10: EXERCISE WITH YOUR PARTNER

Is there anyone who does not wish to lead an active and healthy life? Of course, not! Every single individual loves to be flexible and fit enough to do all their activities independently and enjoy life to the fullest. You must do two things to attain such a life: engage yourself in daily exercise and hang out with your friends or partner. Suppose you get a chance to combine both, i.e., doing workouts along with spending time with your companion. How's the idea? Isn't it exciting? Working out with your buddies will help you feel motivated and also give you a lot of fun. Both you and your partner will feel the urge to fast-track all your fitness goals. Some individuals do exist who love to exercise alone as it helps them to remain focused. But, the case is just the reverse for a maximum number of people. Having a partner for performing exercises boosts their overall performance. Most importantly, you won't feel bored or demotivated for even a single day.

By now, you might have realized what this chapter will deal with. Yes, you will learn about a few essential core exercises you can perform with a single partner or a group of friends. So, let's move ahead!

Russian Twist Using Medicine Ball

This exercise with your partner will act to be a great finisher for targeting your obliques. Every time you twist the torso, obliques are the muscles that will be engaged for a smooth movement. If you and your partner follow this workout regularly, every single corner of your abdominal muscles will become stronger. Those of you who possess the desire to attain a well-toned waistline may perform the Russian twist using a medicine ball. It will also make your back stronger than ever before. The steps are here for a better understanding:

1. To begin this exercise, you and your partner must remain seated back-to-back. Both of you must bend the knees to a small extent and let your heel touch the floor. You and your companion need to lean back by making an angle of almost 45 degrees. Both of your heads will almost stay in touch by maintaining the mentioned angle. The main purpose of leaning backward is to activate your core muscles.

2. You or your friend must begin the workout by holding the medicine ball with both hands. Suppose you are starting the exercise, then you have to grasp the ball close to your chest. After that, your next task is to rotate towards the right side. Once you reach the right, you will be able to transfer the medicine ball to your partner. In the meantime, your partner also has to rotate to his/her left side to receive the ball from your hand.

3. Now, the ball is in the hands of your partner. To transfer it to your hand, he/she needs to rotate the torso all around the right side. Your responsibility will be to twist to the left so that you get to meet your partner and let him/her pass the ball back to you.

4. Both of you must continue revolving and transferring the medicine ball to and fro. You may repeat this exercise a desired number of times or as long as both of you are comfortable. (You must be careful to practice an equal number of repetitions on every single side. It will help in promoting muscle symmetry and also in preventing muscle imbalances. For this, you may either count the number of repetitions you are willing to perform or else

set a timer for each direction.)

High-Five Sit-up

This is a very simple core exercise that you can perform with your partner. For this workout, all you require is a free space on the ground, an exercise mat if you want it, and last but not least, your partner. Doing sit-ups along with high-fives helps to strengthen the external and internal obliques, hip flexors, lower back, and also rectus abdominis. It is a bit more interesting than doing usual sit-ups, as working out with your partner will add fun and variety to this exercise. Increased muscular endurance is a major advantage of this particular exercise. It is also helpful in improving your posture, and a developed posture leads to increased energy, decreased back pain, elevated lung capacity, fewer anxiety headaches, improved digestion and blood circulation, reduced risk of wear and tear, etc. Here are the step-by-step instructions for practicing high-five sit-ups with your workout partner:

1. In the beginning, you need to sit down on the mat or floor by bending your knees. Your feet must remain flat. This is referred to as the sit-up posture. Your partner has to take a similar position, but he/she has to mirror you, that is, stay face to face with you. The toes of your companion must stay in touch with yours. Make sure that the feet of your partner remain hooked underneath your ankles. By doing so, both of you will be able to hold each other securely with the help of body weights.

2. Your next task is lying down and positioning your hands on top of your head. Let your hands touch the back side of your head slightly. This is going to be your beginning position.

3. After this, both of you are supposed to curl the torso and contract the abdominals to rise up simultaneously. When you reach the top position of every single sit-

up, stretch your hands for reaching to your workout partner. Both of you may either touch your fingers or do a high-five.

4. You must make sure that both of you are lowering and rising yourselves at a similar pace. Repeat the steps as long as both of you are comfortable. (Try to squeeze inward as if you are going to create a canoe shape with the help of your abdominals.)

Hip Lifting Plank Hold

Now, this is one of the best workouts for strengthening your glute and core muscles. A plank and hip lift is an ideal combination to work on your core. It activates your oblique muscles as well as assists in developing muscle endurance. You will also be able to toughen and shrink your waistline. Have a look at the steps:

1. At first, deciding who will remain in the standard plank position is necessary. Suppose you choose to do that part in the beginning. Then you need to stay on your hands and hold the plank position.

2. The opposite person, i.e., your partner, has to lie down on the back by placing their legs on you. Now, this is going to add surplus weight to that person who is in the plank position. Thus, it is essential to compress your glutes as well as keep pushing through every single finger.

3. It's time for your partner to perform hip lifts by lifting and lowering their body.

4. After finishing your reps, switch roles and continue.

Various other core exercises do exist that you may perform with your partner, such as butterfly crunches, stacked plank, C-sit squares, Tandem bicycle crunches, V-sit pass, squat-jump together, mountain climbers crunch kiss, stretched leg crunch, etc. You will hopefully enjoy performing different core exercises with your partner. *So, try and have fun!*

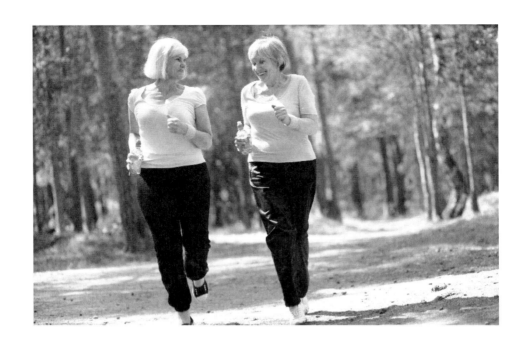

CHAPTER 11: BENEFITS OF DOING CORE EXERCISES WITH A PARTNER

Do you need someone to motivate you to get up at 5:30 or 6:00 a.m. just to practice the core exercises suitable for you? If your answer is yes, then also you need not worry as you are not the only person who faces such challenges as getting up early in the morning and doing workouts. Working together as a team always exhibits affirmative outcomes. The same is the case with doing core exercises too. Not only is performing exercises with a partner or several companions good for enjoying the moment, but it also has a major impact on everyone's health and fitness. In the previous chapter, we dealt with some of the core exercises that can be performed with companions. Here we will discuss the advantages of doing core exercises with your partner. Your partner can be your friends, colleagues, or family members, for example, your siblings, parents, life partner, etc. Selecting a workout partner is completely your personal choice. There is no such strict rule for choosing your partner regarding this matter.

Now, the time has finally arrived to know some detailed information about the benefits of performing core strengthening exercises with your companion.

Healthy Competition

Competition exists in almost all spheres of your life. If you work out with any friend of yours, competition will be present, too, but that would be a healthy one. Such a healthy form of competition will provide both of you with an excellent way to stay fit. For sure, you would not prefer to fall back while exercising with your partner, and vice versa. By exercising together, you will feel the push to give more effort along with being more consistent. When selecting your exercise partner, you just need to be sure that the person you are choosing possesses a similar fitness level like you. Besides helping each other, both of you may compete in simple exercises. This, in turn, will lead to improved stamina and better performance.

No More Quitting

You may not want to get up early in the morning or not feel like hitting the gym after a hectic and tiring day. Sometimes you may feel very lazy or stressed to maintain your workout routine. However, if you have a workout partner, you will surely feel the benefit of being more consistent with your workouts. Both of you will feel the urge to meet with each other and spend some time, even if it is for doing exercises. You will receive motivation from your companion and won't feel like missing or quitting your gym time or workout schedule. It is impossible to reap the full-fledged advantages of core exercise until and unless you do it regularly.

By not quitting your workout routine, you will move one step forward towards achieving your aim of being flexible and strong even in your 60s and 70s.

Reduced Risk of Getting Injured

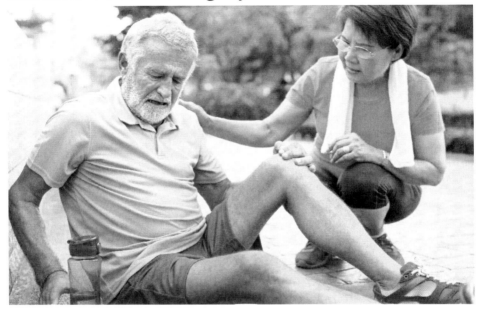

Both you and your companion may help each other during the workout session. Suppose you are doing a plank exercise. If you perform it with your partner, he/she will be able to monitor whether your back is in the right position or not. You need to do the same with your companion by informing them about their position after properly analyzing them. Both of you may convey to each other if anyone is leaning too forward while doing a squat. By doing so, the chances of getting injured will decrease to a great extent. In well-equipped gyms, mirrors are set for solving the same purpose. But, it is not possible to rely completely on mirrors. Thus, this stands to be one of the most fruitful benefits of practicing core exercises with a partner.

Attempting New Workouts

Many people feel frightened and hesitate to try any new exercise-related activities alone as they think they might get injured. If you surround yourself with your workout companions, you will feel less scared to start a new exercise. Having a partner by your side makes it easier to hit free weights, start using gym equipment, or attempt difficult but effective exercises. A similar thing happens when you start following a fresh diet plan and trying out your hands on various exercise equipment. Thus, hanging out with your companions refreshes your mind and helps you be confident about strength training. You must also help your partner so that he/she stops hesitating and take the opportunity to attempt new activities.

Fun-Filled Workout Session

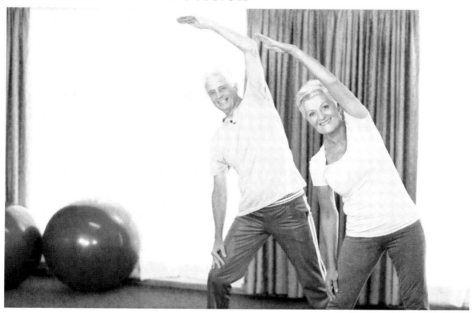

Do you find the gym to be a super boring place? Almost every individual knows the importance of regularly visiting a gym, but at the same time, they also feel bored to keep exercising alone. A treadmill and bench press might not be the perfect means of having an enjoyable time. Going to a gym or doing regular workouts to strengthen your core muscles will become much more enjoyable if you have a workout partner. Even your boring exercise schedule will become filled with fun and laughter. You won't feel bored as you will have someone with whom you can interact in between short breaks. Most importantly, you will also feel the urge to do certain serious exercises with your companions, and that too without being excessively serious. There is no harm in practicing serious activities as well as having fun at the same time. Moreover, it will help in making the environment lighter, which in turn, will let you as well as your partner perform more enthusiastically.

Achieve Your Desired Level of Fitness Faster

You will get the motivation to work harder if you have a workout buddy. You, as well as your companions, will be able to perform various types of exercises together. We all know a common proverb that states, 'unity is strength.' Thus, if you perform together with your exercise partners, all of you will be able to practice even the toughest exercises. By performing together, you will get the opportunity to reach that level of fitness that you always dreamt of, and that too at a faster pace. Your partner can play the role of being your advisor and spotter, and thus your exercise session will become better. It is necessary for you to do the same for your buddy. Both of you may set various fitness goals as well as try accomplishing them together. It is doubtless that you will surely attain outstanding results.

Having Space for Improvement

A huge number of people think that once they have attained their desired fitness goal, there is no room or, rather, no need for further improvement. Do you think in the same manner? If yes, then sorry to say that this thought of yours needs to be changed for a better, stronger, and more flexible future day. When you have your companions to perform exercises with you either in the gym or at home, there always exists space for further development of your physique. There is no end to improvement, and all of you might be aware of the fact that practice makes a man perfect. The more you practice core exercises, the smoother will be your body movements.

If you observe that you have achieved your fitness goal, then also you must not treat this as the ending. Instead of that, set new levels together with your partner and start working to reach that level. Your workout buddy may play the role of an influencer who will teach you various workout regimes for maintaining your core muscles. They can also point out the mistakes that you make while performing the exercises. It will help you a lot to correct those flaws, which will give you more room for progress. Do not forget to help your partner in the same manner.

Receive External Motivation

Are you worrying that you are performing improper exercises? Are you finding certain things to be quite challenging? Are you having a thought of withdrawing your name from the gym? If the response to the questions mentioned above is yes, then all you need is external motivation. Now you might be thinking about where you will get regular motivation. You need not worry at all as your workout partner will help you regarding this matter. He/she will act as an excellent source of consistent motivation. Besides making you feel motivated to take care of your physical well-being, your companion will also enhance your confidence level and keep encouraging you to move forward. With proper motivation, you will not get any sort of negative feelings and also give up the thought of quitting your exercise routine.

Remember to play the same role when your partner feels less motivated. Motivation helps improve a lot as performing exercises with your partner is usually filled up with encouragement. Positive vibes tend to be infectious and have the power to spread like wildfire. Thus, if you practice the exercises with the correct person or the right group, you will surely get uplifted as well as receive encouragement to be your best. Motivation works wonders as it helps people to stick to their wellness and workout routine.

Fitness experts state that you will try to eat well and stay fit if you surround yourself with individuals who are into fitness. Friends or partners are indeed the most valuable assets of a person's life. Having a companion like your workout buddy will never make your exercise schedule dull. One thing that you must consider while choosing your exercise partner is that he/she must also possess similar fitness goals as yours. Now that you are aware of the benefits of doing exercises with a partner, won't you go ahead and choose one? Hopefully, your response will be affirmative.

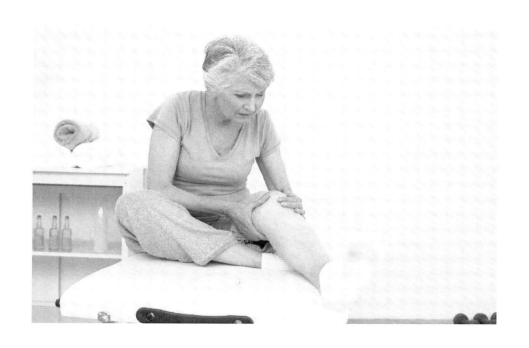

CHAPTER 12: CORE EXERCISES FOR GETTING RELIEF FROM ACHES AND PAINS

Aches and pains have become ever-lasting companions of almost every single individual, especially seniors. Such complications prevent a person from doing all sorts of activities smoothly and easily. Some are there who consume medications to get relief from such pains, such as lower back pain, knee ache, arthritis, or joint pain. Medicines may give you relief, but that is not a permanent solution. Exercise! Yes, one of the most effective and common treatments for treating pain and ache is nothing other than exercise. Depending on your health's current state, regular exercise may enable you to increase mobility, decrease inflammation, minimize overall levels of pain, etc. If you do not have strong core muscles, your entire body will start relying more on the passive structures, like bones and ligaments. This, in turn, will give more stress on the discs, and thus the chances of getting injured or feeling pain will increase.

In this chapter, you will get to know about a few effective core exercises that will not only strengthen and stretch the core muscles but also help relieve aches and pains. *So, here we go!*

Tabletop Leg Press

Often, people refer to this exercise as a 'core connector' as it is an outstanding exercise to engage your core muscles. By doing this exercise, you will get a feeling of what engaging your core actually feels like. Moreover, it is also good for boosting strength and stability. Experts suggest performing this workout after getting up early morning. If senior people practice this exercise regularly and in proper form, it will help them get relief from lower back aches. Want to learn the steps of this pain-relieving core exercise? Here they are:

1. Lie down on the mat or floor by keeping your face in the upward direction. Raise your legs to create a tabletop posture. If in case you are unaware of this position, here is how to make it. You just need to bend your knees at an angle of 90-degree and remain stacked above your hips.

2. After that, your next task is contracting your abdominals to press down your lower back into the ground. Once you are done with this part, crunch upwards for some inches. Then, you are supposed to keep both of your hands in the front portion of your quads.

3. Drive the quads into both your hands. At the same time,

you have to keep pressing them away. Make sure that there must not be any noticeable movement in the body. But it is necessary for you to feel the struggle and also the intense tension inside your core muscles.

4. Lastly, your task is holding this position for a few seconds. You may repeat a desired number of sets.

Glute Bridge

First of all, the glutes bridge will help decrease your lower back ache. Besides working on the glutes, this exercise also works on the lower back, hamstrings, and abdominals. Elderly people won't feel any problem while performing the glute bridge exercise as it does not put any sort of pressure on your lower back. This exercise is also excellent for those who have difficulty doing squats because of hip, knee, or back pain. Stronger glutes will assist in stabilizing the pelvis, and you will be able to remain in the perfect posture from beginning to end. A major reason for suffering from knee pain is not having enough control over the femur. The glutes have the potential to control this leg bone, and thus this workout will also reduce knee pain to a great extent. You will gain the capability of jumping higher and running faster if you practice this workout consistently. Thus, the glutes bridge will provide you with great posture, healthy body movements, and also a back that will be free from discomfort and pain. Let's look at the steps now:

1. To begin with, take the lying down position and bend your feet at right angles. While you are lying down, your heels must be planted strongly on the floor. Your hands will be on either side of your body.

2. After that, squeeze your abdominal muscles and glutes, as well as keep pushing your heels to raise your hips from the floor. Keep lifting until and unless your body creates a straight line between your shoulders and your knees. Next, you have to stay in this posture for a few seconds. While holding this position, you are to make

sure that both your knees remain straight. Do not let them collapse inside.

3. Now, lower your hips very slowly so that you can come back to the beginning position. Repeat as per your comfort.

Reverse Lunge

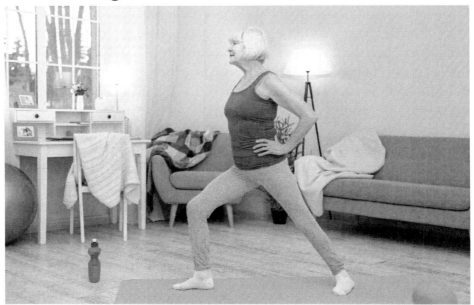

Many people complain that forward lunges hurt their knees a lot. Reverse lunges would be ideal for individuals having knee concerns, little hip mobility, or difficulty in balancing. This exercise helps to activate your glutes, hamstrings, and core. Reverse lunge puts the least stress on the joints. The stability of your legs will also increase if you perform this exercise consistently. This is actually a form of compound exercise which work on multiple muscle groups and joints simultaneously. Besides preventing you from getting injured and giving relief from pains, this workout is helpful in losing more fat. The steps are here for you:

1. Start this exercise by standing straight and keeping a shoulder-width distance between your feet. The next task is to place both your hands either at the back side of your head or on the hip.

2. After that, you have to step backward, say about two feet, with the help of your left foot. While stepping back, make sure to land on your left foot's ball. Your heel must be kept off the floor.

3. Bend both knees so as to create double right angles with the help of your legs.

4. While staying in this position, your shoulders must be directly over your hips. Your chest needs to be upright at the same time. Maintaining a perpendicular distance between the right shin and the floor is necessary. You must not forget to stack the right knee over the right ankle. Engage both your core muscles and butt to create the posture perfectly.

5. Now, your responsibility is to push with the help of the right foot and come back to a standing position.

Lying March

Lying march is an effective exercise to relieve lower back pain. Besides this, it is an excellent way to strengthen your core muscles and lower back. This workout is beneficial in removing excessive pressure from the spinal discs. The process includes the following steps:

1. Lie down on the floor by resting on your back. Bend your knees and place your arms by your side.

2. After that, your next task is tightening the stomach muscles. Lift your left leg very slowly from the ground (approximately three to four inches). Hold this position for a fraction of a second. Then lower your raised body

part on the floor slowly.

3. Once you are done with the left leg, now it's your turn to do the same steps with your right leg. You are to alternate legs and continue 'marching' for almost thirty seconds.

4. You may repeat all the steps for a total number of two or three times.

You may also try out various other core exercises that help in giving relief from lower back aches and pains. A few other exercises include pelvic tilt, planking, partial crunches, hamstring stretches, etc. But before performing the exercises mentioned in this chapter, it would be best to consult with a renowned and experienced physician. He/she will be able to guide you as to which exercises would work best for dealing with the pain that you are suffering from. *Now, it's time to change the page!*

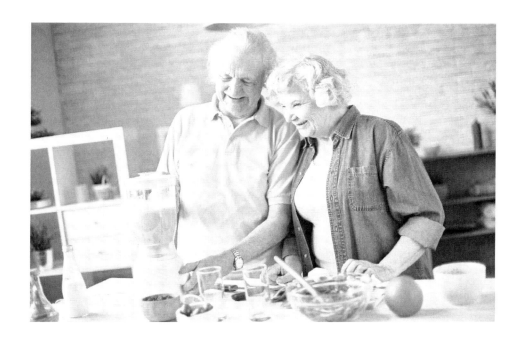

CHAPTER 13: FOODS FOR A STRONGER AND BETTER CORE

While talking about attaining a healthy and fit body, building up strong core muscles has to be the prime objective. It's true that our core is quite complex. As you have reached the end of this book, you might have realized that strengthening your core means working on your abs, muscles surrounding your pelvis, and the back muscles. Performing core exercises regularly will definitely aid in increasing your core strength. Apart from maintaining a consistent workout routine, another highly necessary thing is maintaining a proper diet, including the foods that are helpful for making your core muscles stronger and better. A stronger and toned core will help prevent backaches, build stamina, and let you stay active for longer hours, but it will also help you look great.

Eating the right foods is an integral part of building a healthy core. Here you will come across some of the foods that possess the capability of building a tightened core. All you need to do is purchase such nutritious foods from the nearby market and keep munching throughout the entire day.

Almonds

Now, this is one of the ideal foods that are capable of providing almost all the essential nutrients required by your body. The nutrients present in almonds include protein, fiber, and vitamin E. Almonds also contain magnesium which is vital for maintaining and building muscle tissues. Moreover, it also regulates the level of blood sugar and also produces energy. The almonds' capability to block calories is the most crucial element of creating a lean and strong core. Numerous nutritionists suggest to intake of an ounce of almonds per day, that is, approximately 160 calories. This much almond will help in keeping your abdominal muscles strong and healthy. Other than almonds, you may also consume some other nuts such as walnuts, pecans, Brazil nuts, pistachios, etc. Including seeds in your regular diet, like hemp, pumpkin, flax, chia, etc., will also help build a stronger and healthier core.

Whole Grains

If you are willing to maintain your abs properly, then you need to include whole grains in your daily diet apart from practicing core exercises. Various types of whole grains, such as oats, quinoa, buckwheat, and barley, may prove to be an outstanding addition to the diet. Whole grains are rich in antioxidants, vitamins, and minerals. The most important fact is that whole grains are a great source of fiber, which has the potential to enhance digestion, weight loss, sugar level, and a lot more. Some trustworthy research state that having whole grains may decrease appetite and thus influence the total energy used by your body. Both these factors affect body composition. If you have started aging and are thinking of preparing your body for cheerful future days, you need to incorporate whole grains into your diet and exercise, following the proper steps.

Eggs

Eggs consist of an ideal amino acid balance, which almost every dietitian recommends for this particular reason. You may eat a wholesome breakfast that includes eggs. By doing so, it will lessen all sorts of untimely hunger cravings throughout the entire day. Actually, eggs consist of a perfect combination of fats and proteins, which may effectively satisfy your hunger. If you consume a single egg each day, then it may let you stay away from any sort of unhealthy snacking. This means your chances or cravings for having high-sugar or high-fat foods will be reduced. Therefore, it will help in keeping your core muscles in a proper and desirable shape.

Yogurt

Many people have yogurt without even knowing the actual benefits of including this food item in their diet. Yogurt is referred to as a super healthy food that consists of a sufficient quantity of calcium. This food item is rich in probiotic yogurt, and thus it helps in keeping your digestive system healthier. You might be amazed to know that your core muscles will start strengthening if the problems of gas, constipation, and bloating lower. By eating yogurt regularly, your tummy will appear flat as well as become healthy. A dose of one to three cups of low-fat or fat-free yogurt daily may be great for the midsection. If you feel like changing the taste or adding a little bit of extra fiber, you may combine yogurt with a cup of chopped fresh fruits. Usually, people prefer to have yogurt without any added sugar.

Fresh Fruits and Green Leafy Vegetables

Leafy green veggies are rich in fiber which is helpful in maintaining a slim waistline. Besides this, green vegetables also contain carotenoids, that is essential for improving the immune system and fighting cancers. Almost all types of green veggies possess a rich calcium concentration, which is known to strengthen your muscles. You will also be able to get energy for carrying out energy-draining exercise sessions. Broccoli and spinach are great foods, as one serving of any of these leafy vegetables has the potential to fulfilling twenty percent of the regular fiber requirement.

Just like vegetables, fresh fruits are also rich in nutrients, which means such foods have low calories but higher concentrations of fiber, antioxidants, minerals, and vitamins. People who are looking forward to a diet for building abs must include fruits and vegetables in their diet as these food items boost fat burning and weight loss. While talking about fresh fruits, it is mandatory to talk about apples. Apples consist of almost 85% water and five grams of fiber. Now, this means that if you eat one to two apples regularly, it may help you control unhealthy cravings. Other than this, apples are rich in a compound, namely quercetin, which is useful in fighting cancer and minimizing cholesterol damage. It is also good for your lungs.

So, what are you waiting for? Run to your nearest food market and grab all those foods that will let you strengthen and maintain your core. You must also avoid certain foods which may be harmful to both your waistline and your overall health. Such foods include fried foods, sugar-sweetened drinks, alcoholic beverages, refined grains, sugary snacks, etc. You must never neglect to take proper care of your health and body. Start living happily and healthily even if you have started to grow older. Start believing that age is just a number. *Love yourself! Eat healthy foods! Build up a stronger core! Move with ease!*

CONCLUSION

Thank you for making it through to the end of *Core Exercises for Seniors*. I am pretty sure that you found this book to be quite informative and able to offer helpful tips you need to build up, strengthen, and maintain your core even if you are growing older. Let us also hope that you enjoyed seeking valuable information from this book.

Now that you have stepped into this book's borderline, there is a huge probability that you have come at least one step forward from what you were when you started reading this book. Isn't it so? Suppose you start following the various core exercises that are mentioned here. The outcome is going to be beyond your imagination. We are desirous to help older adults utilize fitness routines as a life-changing tool for prevention and healing, not only for their body but their spirit and mind as well. You need to think young to stay young. Being old does not mean that your life ends there. To bring back the self-confidence of your younger days, taking care of your body, especially your core muscles, is necessary. It is because stronger core muscles are the main element of standing tall with your head held high.

Think of the various symptoms related to aging as a part or chapter of your life. But that does not mean you have to keep lying down and mourn for dealing with the difficulties of aging. By following a consistent exercise regimen, you will be able to fight various types of pain like osteoporosis. If you work your core muscles regularly, you will get the opportunity to keep them healthy and strong. For example, if you perform stability and balance maintaining workouts, you will gain more strength on your feet, and the chances of getting hurt by falling down will gradually decrease. Well, another gift is still left for you. Want to know what's that? Moving the different parts of your body to practice core exercises helps keep the brain sharp, just like in your youth days. So, be smart and sharp and enjoy your aged life. Keep moving! Yes, your body parts. The time has finally come that you must begin practicing the various exercises and the tips for building strength and confidence in your regular life that you have learned from this book.

Finally, if you feel that this book based on ways of being more confident to do your regular chores independently is beneficial for you in any possible way, a brief review on Amazon is always pleasing and treasured!

GLOSSARY

Core: The muscles in the torso, including the abs, back, and hips.

Balance: The ability to maintain equilibrium while standing, walking, or performing other activities.

Posture: The position of the body while sitting, standing, or lying down.

Flexibility: The ability of joints to move through a full range of motion.

Performance: The ability to execute physical tasks efficiently and effectively.

Strength training: A type of exercise that involves resistance to improve muscular strength and endurance.

Cardio: Short for cardiovascular, this refers to exercise that raises the heart rate and improves cardiovascular health.

Muscle imbalances: When one muscle group is stronger or tighter than its opposing muscle group, it can cause postural and movement issues.

Dumbbell: A type of weight that is held in one hand and used for strength training.
Medicine ball: A heavy ball used for strength training and other exercises.

Glutes: Short for gluteal muscles, these are the muscles in the buttocks.

Whole grains: Grains that haven't been processed or refined, such as brown rice or whole wheat bread.

Almonds: A type of nut that is a good source of protein and healthy fats.

Yogurt: A dairy product that is a good source of protein and probiotics

Made in United States
North Haven, CT
24 April 2023

35817507R00059